Practical Nursing and A
for Pupil Nurses

Practical Nursing and Anatomy for Pupil Nurses

Fourth Edition

Jane Forrest SRN, SCM, HV
Margaret Watson RSCN, RGN, RCT

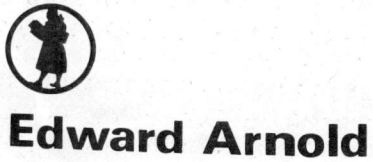

Edward Arnold

©Jane Forrest and Margaret Watson 1981

First published 1966
by Edward Arnold (Publishers) Ltd.
41 Bedford Square, London WC1B 3DQ

Reprinted 1968
Second edition 1969
Reprinted 1970, 1972
Third edition 1974
Reprinted 1976, 1977
Fourth edition 1981
Reprinted 1981

British Library Cataloguing in Publication Data
Forrest, Jane
  Practical nursing and anatomy. — 4th ed.
  1. Practical nursing
  I. Title   II. Watson, Margaret
  610.73   RT62

ISBN 0-7131-4392-4

All Rights Reserved. No part of this publication may be reproduced, stored in a retrieval system, or transmitted in any form or by any means, electronic, mechanical, photocopying, recording or otherwise, without the prior permission of Edward Arnold (Publishers) Ltd.

Set in IBM 11pt Journal by 𝔸 Tek-Art, Croydon, Surrey.
Printed and bound in Great Britain by Pitman Press Ltd, Bath

Preface to the fourth edition

It is with pleasure that I am now able to introduce Miss M. Watson to our many readers as co-author of the fourth edition of this book.

In bringing the contents up to date, I am indebted to her for her valued assistance in revising and amending the text.

To the publishers I am equally grateful for the vast amount of help I have received from them during the past fourteen years.

I hope that nurses will continue to find this book a useful adjunct to their practical training.

JF

Preface to the first edition

The aim of this book is to provide a good foundation of basic facts which will guide the pupil and enrolled nurse to a wider knowledge and understanding of the care of the patient.

Anatomy and Physiology is not treated as a separate, rather dull subject, but is shown to be closely allied to the diseases and treatments which the nurse encounters daily on the wards.

The information contained in the book is presented as simply as possible with explanations of technical terminology given where necessary.

A large number of cross references are given as a further aid to study. Nurses should be encouraged to get into the habit of using the many cross references given as these establish links which connect one fact with another until a complete picture of the subject is obtained.

I sincerely hope that all those pupil nurses embarking on this wonderful career will find this book helpful.

The invaluable suggestions and criticisms of my colleagues during the preparation of the manuscript are gratefully acknowledged.

I am indebted to the publishers for their valued assistance, particularly to the late Mr. T. H. Clare and to Miss B. Koster.

Acknowledgement of permission to reproduce figures is due to William Heinemann Medical Books Ltd., (Fig. 13), The Royal Life Saving Society United Kingdom, (Fig. 94), the Scholl Mfg. Co. Ltd. (Fig. 101), and to the St. John Ambulance Association, The St. Andrew's Ambulance Association and the British Red Cross Society. (Fig. 98-100, 102 and 103 from *Authorised Nursing Manual*).

JF

Contents

1. **The nurse** — 1
   Personal hygiene — 2
   Professional etiquette — 3
   The approach to the patient — 3
   Noise — 4
   Writing ward reports — 6

2. **Cleanliness of the ward and annexes** — 7
   The ward kitchen — 7
   The ward bathroom and sluices — 7

3. **Hospital beds and bedding** — 9
   Making the patient's bed — 10
   Equipment used for the comfort of the patient — 11
   Special beds — 12
   Positions used in nursing — 13

4. **Care of the patient** — 15
   Admission of patients — 15
   Discharge and transfer of the patient — 17
   Observation of the patient — 18
   Rigor — 24
   The pulse — 26
   Respiration — 27
   Faeces — 27
   Suppositories — 29
   Enemata — 30
   Rectal washout — 32
   Treatment of flatus — 32
   Colostomy washout — 34
   Caecostomy — 34

5	**The skin**	36
	The formation and function of the skin	36
	Care of the skin	37
	Care of the scalp and hair	40
	Pressure sores	42
	Diseases of the skin	45
	Common disorders of the skin	46
	Starch poultice	49
6	**The respiratory system**	50
	Common respiratory diseases	52
	Inhalations	56
	Administration of oxygen	57
7	**The heart and circulation**	59
	Haemorrhage	63
	Some common diseases of the heart and blood vessels	66
	Measurement of blood pressure	69
8	**The blood**	71
	Blood grouping and transfusion	72
	Some common diseases of the blood	73
	Inflammation	74
	Hot applications	75
	Cold applications	76
9	**The urinary system**	77
	Urine testing	80
	Intake and output charting	82
	Catheterization	83
	Some common diseases of the urinary system	86
10	**Food, diets and digestion**	89
	Food	89
	The digestive system	93
	The digestive process	101
	Feeding the patient	102
	Diets	104
	Disorders of the digestive system	106
	Artificial feeding	109

11	**The lymphatic system**	112
	Functions of the lymphatic system	112
	Hodgkin's disease	114
	The spleen	114
12	**The endocrine glands**	115
	The pituitary gland	115
	The thyroid gland	116
	The parathyroid glands	117
	The thymus gland	118
	The adrenal glands	118
	The islets of Langerhans	118
	The sex glands	118
13	**Administration of medicines**	119
	Legislation	119
	Administration of medicines	119
	Intramuscular injections	121
	Hypodermic injections	123
	Intravenous injections	123
	Intravenous infusions	124
	Classification of drugs	124
14	**Micro-organisms and infection**	126
	Bacteria	127
	Aspects of infectious diseases	127
	Infectious diseases	132
15	**Disinfection and sterilization. Surgical nursing**	136
	Disinfection	136
	Sterilization of equipment	137
	Surgical nursing	138
	Ward dressings	140
16	**Tissues of the body**	150
	Cells and tissues	150
17	**The muscular system**	153
	Voluntary muscles	153
	Involuntary muscles	155
	Cardiac muscle	155
	Disorders affecting muscle tissue	155

18	**The brain and the nervous system**	157
	The cerebrum	158
	The cerebellum	158
	The pons varolii	159
	The medulla oblongata	159
	The autonomic or sympathetic nervous system	160
	Common diseases of the brain	161
	Common diseases affecting the nervous system	165
19	**The eye**	168
	The eyelids	168
	The lacrimal glands	168
	The eyeball	168
	The lens	169
	Some disorders of the eye	170
	Nursing treatment of the eye	171
20	**The ear**	174
	The outer ear	174
	The middle ear	174
	The inner ear	175
	Hearing	176
21	**The skeleteon**	177
	Bone structure	177
	The skeleton	179
	Diseases of bones and joints	190
	Injuries to bones and joints	193
22	**The reproductive system**	202
	Male reproductive organs	202
	Female reproductive organs	203
	Gynaecological procedures	204
23	**Care of the elderly and chronically ill patient**	206
	Geriatric nursing	206
	The chronically ill patient	209
24	**Burns, diabetes, neoplasms, tuberculosis, venereal diseases, last offices**	210
	Burns	210
	Diabetes mellitus	211
	Neoplasms	215
	Tuberculosis	216

	Venereal diseases	218
	Last offices	220
25	**The normal baby**	223
	The child in hospital	224
	Infant feeding	227
	The older child	229
	Safety in the children's ward	230
26	**First aid treatment in emergencies**	232
	General rules of first aid	232
	First aid treatments	234
	Poisons	239
	Artificial respiration	239
	Other emergencies	243
	Bandaging	245
	Index	252

1
The nurse

When prospective nurses enter hospital for the first time for training, they enter a different world to that to which they have become accustomed, whether at home, at school or in some other occupation. In hospital they will find themselves working with people of different classes, creeds, temperaments and professional status, but all with one objective in view; the care and comfort of the patient and the relief of suffering. It is for this that nurses are training, and to this end they should develop those qualities necessary to become well-trained and efficient nurses.

Good nurses are kindly, courteous and considerate, without familiarity, either with patients or senior staff. They are cheerful, observant and helpful, and are willing to undertake any task they may be asked to perform. For meals, duty and lectures they are punctual always, and their loyalty is such that they can be trusted implicitly in the small, as well as in the important matters and for this, self-discipline must be developed.

In order that nurses may remain interesting and interested people, they should endeavour to maintain lively curiosity in events and activities outside the hospital; in books, daily papers, and in other people and their achievements. The nurse who can talk of nothing but hospital life becomes a dull companion. The mind becomes stagnant, and boredom and irritability may result, to the detriment of both nurse and patient.

Life in hospital is essentially communal and, in their relationships with their colleagues, nurses should be friendly and tolerant. In any community the most popular person is the one who exhibits a good-natured, non-critical attitude towards other people, thus creating a pleasant atmosphere at all times.

Nursing is the finest and most worthwhile profession, which brings its own reward to the enthusiastic pupil, yet no one can deny that it is hard work, especially during the first few months when everything seems so strange. Personal health should be one of the first considerations, and in this matter nurses have a duty to themselves which must not be neglected, otherwise they will be unable to give of their best to their patients. Certain health rules must be observed if a good standard of fitness is to be maintained.

An average of eight hours' sleep is needed to relieve the mental and physical wear and tear of a busy day. It is during sleep that body tissues are rebuilt and repaired, especially those of the important nervous system.

The diets planned by hospital caterers and dietitians include all the necessary food factors for the maintenance of good health. Meals are served regularly and in sufficient quantity for the needs of the body, but for non-resident nurses, care should be taken that nourishing meals are available at regular intervals. No meals should be missed.

Nurses are often heard to say that they 'get enough exercise on the wards'. This is wrong thinking. Exercise should be taken outdoors in the open air, away from the wards, so that the blood may obtain a fresh supply of oxygen. Lack of fresh air causes tiredness and lethargy.

Smoking is a serious health hazard and nurses should set an example by refraining and encouraging others to stop the habit. Stale smoke on clothes and breath can be very unpleasant, particularly to a sick patient.

Personal hygiene

The nurse is constantly on her feet and care should be taken to ensure the feet do not become sore or blistered. It is a good plan to have two pairs of shoes, to be worn on alternate days. A daily bath or shower should be taken and tights changed daily. The advice of a chiropodist should be sought if necessary.

As well as a daily bath, suitable deodorants should be used. No trace of body odour should be noticeable. Any rashes or other abnormalities of the skin which occur should receive appropriate attention.

Care should be taken of the skin of the hands. Cuts or scratches should be treated at once and kept covered to avoid risk of infection. Nails should be clean and short: long fingernails may injure the patient. Nail varnish must not be worn when on duty as varnish tends to flake off and may cause infection.

The nurse must present a well-groomed appearance. Uniform should be clean and neat and no jewellery nor wristwatches should be worn with uniform. Hair should be clean and tidy and off the collar.

Professional etiquette

By this is meant the code of behaviour expected of a nurse. It represents a high standard which each nurse endeavours to maintain all through a nursing career. This needs discipline in matters of behaviour. It is for this reason that hospital rules are evolved, to guide the pupils in their training so that they may be respected by all with whom they come into contact, outside, as well as inside the hospital. Etiquette implies courtesy and the courteous nurse will have little difficulty in carrying out the rules which are observed in all hospitals.

The approach to the patient

Nursing is a career in which human relationships are the most important factors. The basis of all good nursing lies in such attributes as kindness, courtesy and efficiency, without which a nursing career would be impossible.

Patients are people and it must be remembered that each occupant of a hospital bed has a life outside the ward, a fact which nurses tend to overlook in their preoccupation with hospital duties. There may be anxieties concerning the family, or personal problems which may harass the patient's mind, yet rarely will the nursing staff hear of these worries and anxieties. Too often they are repressed, to the detriment of progress of the patient, unless nurses are observant and have the ability to communicate their sympathetic understanding.

Lack of privacy in the ward is one of the most trying factors in a patient's life, particularly in regard to such things as washings, bathings, toilet rounds and the many other routine procedures. To the nurse these things are a normal part of life in a general ward, but they are *not* regarded in such a matter-of-fact way by the patient, who may be longing for the seclusion of home.

Sympathetic nurses will understand this point of view and will do all that is possible to make the patient feel at ease by preventing any undue exposure or publicity. They will treat the patient as an individual and not as another 'case', thus helping to retain the self-confidence which illness or injury may undermine or destroy. In these days we know that the mind does influence the body and that the manner in which the patient is approached by other people has an effect on progress and recovery.

On admission to the ward, the new patient should be greeted

4   Practical nursing

with a reassuring and cheerful manner, which will go far in giving confidence and in making the hospital seem a less frightening place, especially to those who feel extremely nervous and apprehensive.

The average sick person shows an extraordinary courage in the face of pain and trouble, but occasionally we meet the unhappy, complaining type of patient. It is with these unfortunate people that all the resources of the nurse are called upon. An attempt should be made to understand the reason for such behaviour, remembering that worry, pain or fear may be the underlying cause. Patience, humour and sympathy are needed to overcome the mental distress so often resulting in apparent irritability.

When carrying out nursing procedures, do not presume that the patient knows what is about to happen. Remember that, to the patient, hospital routine is strange and may give rise to unnecessary fears. The patient should not be left unattended behind screens; always explain why the screens are drawn, even if only for a blanket bath. A few seconds spent in explanation and reassurance will relieve any feeling of anxiety and may mean a great deal to the patient.

Many patients find it difficult to sleep whilst in hospital and the nights seem very long to a sick person. It is the nurse's duty to see that everything possible is done to overcome this and to make the patient comfortable. Here again, it may be found that mental distress, or worry of some kind, is preventing the complete relaxation so essential for the promotion of sleep. A few sympathetic words may bring reassurance and a happier state of mind to the patient who realizes that someone is aware of the inability to rest. The sense of loneliness from which many people suffer during the night, especially when in strange surroundings, is lessened by the attention of an observant nurse.

Noise

It has become increasingly evident that inescapable noise such as that produced by aircraft, road traffic, industrial machinery, etc. has a detrimental effect on the nervous system of many people, especially those living or working in or around the larger towns and cities.

The elimination, or at least the lessening, of noise is now a major problem to which scientists, engineers, architects and the medical profession are giving a great deal of consideration.

This problem is one that particularly affects hospitals, and in the newer hospital buildings every effort is being made to overcome it with the use of special insulating material, flooring, double glazing, etc.

All this is being carried out to ensure that sick people are not unduly disturbed. But what of the noise in the ward and its environs?

Noise in the hospital ward is unnerving and devastating to the patient, especially if the patient is helpless, seriously ill or newly admitted and therefore unused to hospital routine. Few patients will complain of noise. Many are 'afraid of being a nuisance' or say they 'did not want to bother the nurses' — a statement that should never be necessary. People do not need to be very ill to be actuely aware of noise.

All nurses who have been on night duty know the agony of being kept awake during the day, when they should be sleeping, by noise made by unthinking colleagues who are themselves either on day duty or off duty. How much more distress it must cause a patient who cannot escape from a noisy ward. The alert, intelligent nurse will be well aware of this problem and will make every effort to keep the ward as quiet as possible.

Hospital kitchens are invariable adjacent to the ward, where the noise of clattering cutlery and crockery can be heard clearly. All doors between the kitchens and wards should be kept closed whilst meal trolleys are being cleared, to lessen the noise impact. Squeaking wheels on trolleys, beds and other wheeled furniture should be swiftly dealt with: an oil can is small enough to be readily available. It takes but a moment of time to rectify such irritating and excruciating noises. Chairs without castors should be *lifted* from one place to another, never dragged across the floor.

Difficulties may arise where unrestricted visiting is the rule. Too many visitors around the beds invariably raises the level of noise in the ward. People tend to forget that there may be very ill patients in the beds a few yards away. Children should not be allowed to run up and down the ward at will or to make any undue noise unchecked. During visiting hours, the nursing staff should be alert to the conditions prevailing in the ward, especially to the degree of noise at any time. Most visitors will comply with a firm, courteous request for less noise.

A nurse should never raise her voice above normal level. Even when dealing with a deaf patient, communication can be established without the need to shout. Slow, clear enunciation combined with gestures is usually sufficient to convey understanding.

During the day a reasonable amount of noise may be tolerable: noise cannot be eliminated entirely, but at night every small sound seems to be magnified so that a patient on the verge of sleep will immediately become fully awake. Most sounds can be muffled at night and the good night nurse will do everything possible to ensure that the ward is kept quiet.

One of the most irritating sounds to a patient trying to sleep is the sibilant hiss of whispering voices in the immediate vicinity of the ward, which, if continued for any length of time, can prove distressing and result in hours of lost sleep.

Every nurse on the hospital staff can play her part in keeping noise to a minimum in the nurses' residence and in the hospital.

Writing ward reports

The aim of giving and receiving reports is to maintain an unbroken chain of communication between all nursing and medical staff so that no aspect of the treatment and condition of the patient is overlooked. Good reporting depends on good observation. The Kardex system of reporting is used in most hospitals, but whichever method is adopted, the basic information remains much the same.

Reports must be written in ink for legibility and durability because they are filed for future reference. Medical abbreviations should not be used; these can lead to confusion and mistakes. The report should be written concisely and to the point but information so given must be accurate. Where there is the slightest doubt, the nurse should check a statement *before* putting it into writing. All reports must be signed. In the event of legal proceedings a signature may be required in a court of law.

Meaningless phrases such as 'condition satisfactory' should be avoided. These are non-specific. No personal comments may be written into a report; nurses must report exactly what they observe and not what they feel about a patient. Any special incidents, e.g. accident or injury to a patient, must be reported. In addition, it is usually necessary to fill out a special accident form.

In addition to reports on each patient, ward reports are written, usually twice daily, and sent to the nursing administration department. The content varies from hospital to hospital but this usually includes information on numbers of admissions, discharges and deaths, and a brief account of any severely ill patients.

2
Cleanliness of the ward and annexes

The cleanliness of the ward and annexes is under the control and supervision of the domestic supervisor in liaison with the ward sister. The nurse must ensure that the patient is disturbed as little as possible and should be available to advise and assist with moving of the patients and special equipment. Local policies vary, but frequently the nursing staff are responsible for damp dusting equipment attached to patients, particularly in intensive care areas. At all times patient safety is the responsibility of the nurse.

The ward kitchen

Nurses must assist in maintaining cleanliness of the ward kitchen by ensuring that all equipment is put away in its proper place. All crockery and cutlery should be inspected before being taken to the bedside. Utensils for infectious patients should ideally be disposable but, if not, must be sterilized after use.

Nurses must acquaint themselves with the local policy regarding the return of unused food and the disposal of waste food.

The ward bathroom and sluices

Sluices and lavatories should always be ready for use, in spotless condition. All articles should be cleaned and put away in the proper place after use. In general, the nursing staff are responsible for the cleanliness of articles used by the patient at the bedside, i.e. bedpans, urinals, tooth mugs, wash bowls. Domestic staff will clean the toilets and bathrooms daily, but the nurse must ensure that the baths are cleaned after each patient has used them.

Nurses must familiarize themselves with the local policy for the disposal of rubbish, sharps (i.e. sharp objects), soiled and infected linen and other contaminated articles.

8   Practical nursing

Most sluice rooms now have bedpan washers and sterilizers. Where these are not available, bedpans must be thoroughly cleaned after use and soaked in disinfectant daily.

3
Hospital beds and bedding

The hospital bed is so constructed that it can be easily cleaned and disinfected when required. The bedstead is fitted with large, rubber castors which allow the bed to be moved with ease, and a special braking attachment prevents it from moving when in position in the ward. The height of the bed is such that the patient may receive attention without undue fatigue on the part of the nurses, at the same time allowing the floor under the bed to be seen and cleaned easily.

Mattresses may be made of sponge rubber or with internal springs. All mattresses are protected with a plastic covering.

Pillows used for supporting the patient may be filled with horsehair or flock, whilst those under the head are filled with sponge rubber or feathers for comfort. Where necessary, the pillow may be protected by a plastic cover placed underneath the pillow-case.

Drawsheets are made of strong cotton or twill because they need to stand a great deal of hard wear. The drawsheet is often placed under the buttocks and can be changed easily and as often as required, without undue disturbance of the patient. The use of drawsheets with patches or darns should not be allowed, as they will cause the patient pain or discomfort and may be the cause of bed sores.

Draw mackintoshes are now made of plastic and are used under the drawsheet. The top edge of the draw mackintosh and sheet should be at the lower level of the pillows. Drawsheets and mackintoshes are used for incontinent and very ill patients.

Sheets are usually made of cotton. Linen is very cold to the touch. Counterpanes are also made of cotton as they need to be washed frequently.

Blankets may be made of wool but these have been largely superseded by covers made of a cellular cotton material which is light in weight and can be boiled, both of which are advantages not found with woollen blankets, especially in the prevention of cross infection in the ward.

10 Practical nursing

Thinner blankets or flannelette sheets are used for placing next to the patient in bed for extra warmth, or for blanket bathing. Coloured blankets are used for admission beds, for patients sitting out of bed or attending departments outside the ward, such as x-ray or physiotherapy. All bedding is expensive and should be treated with the utmost care. No torn linen should be used in bedmaking but should be put out for repair.

Making the patient's bed

The primary aim in bed-making is to make the patient as comfortable as possible. Two nurses should make an occupied bed together, working smoothly without undue disturbance of the patient. One nurse working by herself is a waste of time and is far more exhausting for the patient.

General principles for bed-making

All clean linen required and a receptacle for soiled linen should be collected before the bed is stripped.

As the folded bedding is removed, it is placed over a bed-stripper, or on two chairs placed back to back at the foot of the bed.

Bed-clothes must not be allowed to touch the floor or they will become contaminated by bacteria which exist in dust, thus spreading infection.

Nearby windows should be closed to avoid chilling the patient.

Nurses must work quickly and quietly, with no unnecessary talking between them.

Each article of bedding is removed separately, folded into three, concertina-wise, and placed on the chairs.

Bedding should not be shaken as this spreads dust and bacteria.

Care should be taken that the mattress is not banged into position when making an occupied bed. This may cause pain or distress to the patient.

A blanket must be left next to the patient when stripping the bed and the top sheet slipped out from under it.

All creases or crumbs must be brushed out from under the patient and the bottom sheet and drawsheet pulled taut and the ends tucked firmly under the mattress.

Pillows are removed, shaken up and replaced, making sure

they are in the correct position for the patient's comfort. The open ends of the pillows should face away from the direction of the ward door. The completed bed should look tidy, with neat corners, and with the patient in the correct position for comfort and good nursing. In particular, the top clothes should be loose to allow movement and prevent foot-drop. Before leaving the bedside, the nurses must make sure that the patient is comfortable with everything needed within reach.

The appearance of the ward depends a great deal on the way the beds are made. Linen should be immaculate, counterpanes put on with care and beds left in a straight line, with all castors turned inwards, giving a look of efficiency to the whole ward. Napkins should be used at meal times to prevent soiling of linen.

Equipment used for the comfort of the patient

For the added comfort of the patient, special equipment is used according to the type of nursing required.

Bed cradles made of metal are used to take the weight of the bed-clothes from the body. When in use, a lightweight blanket is placed over the patient for warmth.

Bed rests help to support the patient. They are often part of the bed-head and can be adjusted as required, or they may be portable. These are made of wood or tubular steel with canvas strips to support the pillows and which fold flat when not in use.

Air rings are hollow, rubber rings fitted with a valve. These are blown up to form a cushion on which the patient sits to prevent pressure sores at the lower part of the back. Rings may also be made of sponge rubber. All rings must be put into a cotton cover before being placed under the patient.

Fracture boards are placed underneath the mattress to prevent it sagging when a patient is in a plaster splint or needs firm support after spinal injuries or operations.

Sandbags are used to support or immobilize some part of the body such as a fractured pelvis.

Bed blocks are used to raise the head or the foot of the bed by resting the castors in the cup-like depressions in the tops of the blocks. These are used in cases of shock or haemorrhage. the bed can also be raised by means of metal elevators which may either be attached to the bed or may be portable.

Practical nursing

Special beds

Admission or emergency bed

The bottom of the bed is made up as usual, as far as the drawsheet, with one pillow on a chair at the side of the bed. The bed is then covered with an admission blanket which is turned over at the sides and tucked in. The second, coloured admission blanket is folded lengthwise and placed on top. The rest of the bedclothes are folded into a pack which is placed on the bed, over the admission blankets.

Fracture bed

This is made as for the emergency bed, with the addition of fracture boards underneath the mattress. A cradle, towel and sandbags should be placed in readiness to protect and control the site of the fracture. Bed blocks may be needed where extensions are to be applied.

Plaster bed

This is made in the same way as a fracture bed, with the addition of a small blanket to cover the patient, an extra pillow protected with a plastic cover on which to rest the limb and a sock to cover the exposed toes of the patient. If this is done, the toes must be inspected regularly to check the colour and for the presence of any swelling. After plaster of Paris has been applied, a cradle is placed over the plaster and the lower end of the bed left open until the plaster is dry.

Divided or amputation bed

The bed is made up with two sets of top bed-clothes, one over the upper half and one over the lower half of the patient, so that the stump of the amputated limb is visible to the nursing staff, in case of haemorrhage. The stump can be seen at the point where the two sets of bedclothes meet. A blanket is placed next to the patient for warmth. Other equipment needed will be a dressing mackintosh and towel to be placed under the stump, a towel and two sandbags to keep it in position, bed blocks in case of haemorrhage and a tourniquet fastened to the foot of the bedstead, out of sight of the patient.

Hospital beds and bedding 13

Operation bed

The bottom of the bed is made up in the ordinary way. A small mackintosh and anaesthetic towel is placed over the mattress at the head of the bed in case the patient vomits on return from the theatre. The top bed-clothes are folded lengthwise into a pack and placed on top of the bed. Bed blocks and oxygen should be in readiness by the bedside. A vomit bowl and tissues and resuscitation equipment should be at hand.

Positions used in nursing

The position in which the patient is nursed depends on the disease, the symptoms and the treatment, and it has an important bearing on progress and recovery. (See Fig. 3.1).

Recumbent position
The patient lies flat in the bed with one pillow to ensure complete rest.

Semi-recumbent position
Two or three pillows are placed under the head; this position is often adopted during convalescence.

Upright position
The patient is propped up in the sitting position and is supported by a bed rest and pillows. A sandbag or foot board is placed at

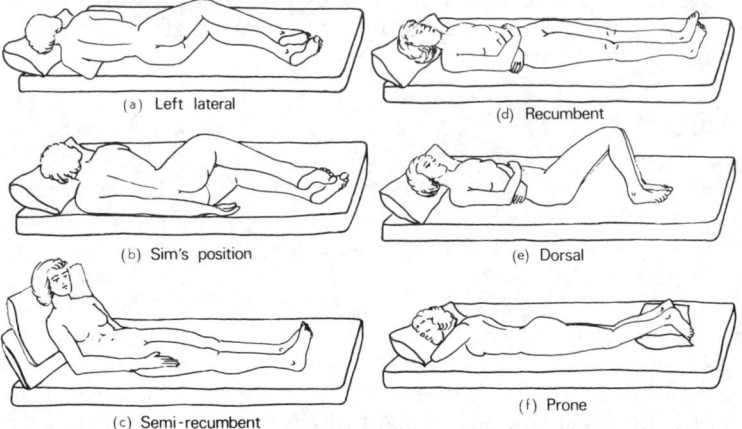

(a) Left lateral
(b) Sim's position
(c) Semi-recumbent
(d) Recumbent
(e) Dorsal
(f) Prone

Fig. 3.1 Positions used in nursing.

the foot of the bed to prevent the patient from slipping down the bed. The patient should be encouraged to move the legs where allowed, in order to prevent thrombosis. This position has several advantages, it allows efficient drainage after abdominal operations, assists breathing in severe respiratory or cardiac disease and, postoperatively, encourages personal interest in the activities of the ward. A patient sitting upright usually feels much better than when lying flat in the bed.

Left lateral position
The patient lies on the left side with the buttocks on the edge of the bed and the knees drawn upwards. One pillow is placed under the head.

Sim's position
This is an exaggerated form of the left lateral position. The patient lies with the head and chest resting on a pillow, with the left arm lying behind the back. The knees are flexed, the right knee more so than the left. This position is usually adopted for vaginal examination.

Dorsal position
The patient is placed on the back with the knees raised for abdominal examination, or when giving vaginal treatments.

Prone position
The patient lies face downward with the head turned to one side. A pillow placed under the ankles prevents pressure of the toes on the mattress. This position may be used after operation or injury to the back.

4
Care of the patient

Admission of patients

Patients are admitted to the wards from a waiting list, as emergencies, or they may have been written for as special cases. In many instances the patient arrives nervous and ill at ease, and it is the nurse who is given the opportunity of extending a courteous, cheerful and reassuring welcome. When the patient is accompanied by a relative or friend, that person also should be treated with the same courtesy and consideration. In no instance should the patient be given the impression of being 'just another case', or that the nurse is too busy to be able to spare much time. Nor should the relatives feel that they are being a nuisance: they should be offered a chair and asked to wait until the patient is settled in the ward. The ward sister is always notified of impending admissions, but should be informed of the arrival of a new patient.

Particulars to be taken by the nurse are as follows.
Name and address of the patient.
Age and date of birth.
Occupation or school.
Sex; whether married, single or widowed.
Religion and name of the patient's minister of religion.
Name and address of nearest relative (with the telephone number).
Name of the home doctor.
Name of the medical officer in charge of the case.
The date and time of admission.

In hospitals where the nursing process has been implemented, a proper nursing history is taken.

When all the particulars have been completed, the patient is taken to the bedside, introduced to the other patients, shown how to store personal belongings in the locker and shown where the bathrooms and toilets are situated.

A consent form for operation or anaesthetic must be signed

by the patient if an adult, or by the next of kin if the patient is under age or is in any way incapable of signing. This is the responsibility of the doctor who must first explain the nature of the operation or treatment.

The temperature, pulse and respirations are taken and recorded and a specimen of urine should be obtained and tested. The result of this test must also be recorded. An identification bracelet is attached to the patient's wrist. Details should be checked by the patient or a relative.

When the patient is comfortably in bed, the relatives may be escorted to the bedside to say good-bye, but they must not be allowed to leave the hospital until interviewed by the ward sister or deputy, who will give them any information they may require.

In the case of seriously ill or unconscious patients, valuables or documents must be checked in the presence of the patient or relatives, listed, checked by another nurse and handed to sister for safe keeping. The patient's clothing is sent home if possible, or, if no relatives are present, the clothing is listed, labelled with the patient's name and stored until called for.

Instructions regarding a bath must be obtained from the senior nursing staff. If necessary, the patient is bathed, but this is usually quite unnecessary and demoralizing. The patient may have a bath before bedtime.

Emergency admissions brought in by ambulance or admitted from casualty are put straight into bed and blanket bathed if necessary. The presence of any scars, rashes or deformities should be noted.

Admission of children and infants

The procedure is the same as when admitting adults, but more effort is usually required to reassure the child, whose confidence must be gained. It is a mistake to show signs of haste or impatience, or to attempt to undress and bath the child immediately on admission. A small child who becomes very frightened on admission, by finding himself in a strange place, surrounded by unfamiliar faces and who sees his mother apparently deserting him, will be lonely and miserable, and may suffer from the effects of this experience for many years. The mother should be invited to stay throughout the admission procedure. The temperature, pulse and respirations are recorded. The identity bracelet must be carefully checked by the mother before attaching it to the child's wrist or ankle. The child should be shown where his bed and locker are situated and then introduced to the other children in the ward and also the play lady.

It is usually quite unnecessary to bath and put to bed a child admitted from the waiting list. Many children associate bed with punishment and cannot understand why they should go to bed when feeling perfectly well.

All this requires a good deal of time, but it is well spent, because the child will feel that the hospital is a friendly place and will settle down much more quickly. Parents should be advised to bring a favourtie toy to be left with the child: this forms a familiar link with home and may lessen the sense of loss from which most children suffer during their first few days in hospital. Many hospitals now have facilities for mothers to live in, and the mothers should be encouraged to do so, particularly if their child is under 5 years of age.

Additional information is required from the parent when admitting children and a consent form for anaesthetic, operation, or blood transfusion must be signed if necessary.

Additional particulars required are listed below.

Address of parents if different from the child's.

Religion, and whether the child has been christened or not. (Where children have not been christened, the wishes of the parents must be ascertained with regard to this, so that the correct minister of religion may be notified if necessary).

What infectious diseases the child has had.

Whether the child has been in contact with infection during the preceding three weeks.

Whether the child has been immunized or vaccinated, against what diseases and when.

When a baby is admitted, still further information is needed.

The type and amount of food the baby is having.

The times at which feeds are due.

The weight of the baby and the average weekly loss or gain.

Breast-feeding mothers should be offered accommodation in the hospital.

Discharge and transfer of the patient

When a patient is to be discharged to his home, the relatives are notified one or two days beforehand of the date and time at which they may call for him, bringing his clothes if they have been sent home. Personal belongings are returned to him just before he is due to leave and a receipt obtained for any valuables or documents which may have been kept in safe custody.

Instruction will be given to the patient and/or the relatives as to the date and time of any appointments made for him in the out-patient department or clinic. Any special instructions regarding, for example, medicines to be taken or limitations of activity, must be clearly given also. The patient should be escorted from the ward either by a nurse or a porter and seen safely off the premises.

Where a patient is to be transferred to another hospital he should be told when and why he is going so that any undue anxiety may be allayed. The relatives should be informed in advance of the impending transfer or, if this is not possible, at the earliest opportunity.

Immediately a patient is discharged or transferred, the bed is stripped and the linen and blankets sent to the laundry. Disposable waterproof sheeting is destroyed; others are washed, disinfected, dried and stored on rollers. The bed, locker and bed table, if not returned to a central area, must be washed and left to air and the bed then made up with clean linen. All nursing notes and charts must be carefully filed in the patient's case folder.

Observation of the patient

An essential part of the nurse's training is the development of the power of observation. The ability to notice and to *report accurately* any unusual sign, symptom or change in the condition of the patient, is the hallmark of the efficient nurse. It is on these observations and reports that the senior staff rely in the treatment, and sometimes the diagnosis, of the patient. The doctor is not always present in the ward to see how the patient is progressing, but must rely on the nursing staff for this information. It is not necessary to stand at the bedside of the patient in order to know what is happening. Observant nurses note every small detail, even whilst apparently busy with other duties: they are never so absorbed that the patient is forgotten. Eyes, ears and brain, as well as the hands, are constantly alert so that nurses are aware of all that takes place in their wards.

Observations to be made will include the following.

Expression. Much may be deduced from the patient's face; fear, anxiety, pain or approaching collapse may be noted in facial expression.

Colour. The face may be blue (cyanosis), often associated with respiratory or heart diseases; pale as in shock, yellow as in jaundice or flushed, indicating a high temperature.

Attitude. The position in which the patient lies may indicate pain or discomfort in some part of the body.

Temperature, may vary from day to day.

Pulse rate, which may also vary and is an important guide to the condition of the patient.

Respirations, of which there are several types, each having a bearing on the condition of the patient.

Skin may appear dry, scaly, moist or erupting.

Urine. The amount, colour and constituents are noted and recorded.

Faeces. The colour, constituents and consistency should be observed (see p. 27).

Vomiting. Colour, consistency, odour and time of vomiting should be noted, particularly in relation to taking of food and drink.

(*a*) *Vomited blood* (*haematemesis*) appears as dark brown granules due to the action of the digestive juices on blood which is escaping into the stomach. This type of vomit is known as 'coffee ground vomit' owing to the resemblance to coffee grounds.

(*b*) *Greenish fluid* may be due to the presence of bile.

(*c*) *Dark brown faecal* vomit is a serious sign and may be due to intestinal obstruction.

(*d*) *Bright red blood* in the vomit may be the result of bleeding from the back of the nose, throat or tongue.

In addition to these observations, the presence or absence of pain during an attack of vomiting should be noted, whether the pain was relieved or not, or whether vomiting was forcible. (This type of vomiting is known as 'projectile' in which the vomited material is thrown for some distance and is a serious sign of obstruction of some part of the upper digestive tract.)

Nausea is a feeling of sickness without actual vomiting.

Sputum is a sticky fluid expelled from the respiratory organs by coughing, and may have the following appearances:

    (*a*) *rusty-coloured streaks,* typical of pneumonia;

    (*b*) *mucoid, white or yellowish,* occurs in bronchitis;

    (*c*) *purulent, containing pus,* as in some cases of lung abscess or tuberculosis;

    (*d*) *blood stained, bright red and frothy.* This may be due to haemorrhage in the lungs (haemoptysis) and must be reported at once. The patient is often very frightened, needs reassurance, and must not be left alone.

20 Practical nursing

Sputum is loaded with bacteria and a watch must be kept so that the disposable sputum cartons do not become too full. The lids should be put on very securely before disposal. Where a specimen of sputum is required for pathological examination, the patient is given a special sterile flask in which to collect the specimen. This should be obtained in the morning, before the patient takes anything by mouth.

Cough is caused by irritation of the respiratory passage. The nurse should observe the type of cough, whether dry, moist, accompanied by pain or spasm, or whether aggravated by movement on the part of the patient.

Hiccough is due to spasm of the diaphragm. It should be noted whether it is continuous or intermittent. Continuous hiccough is a serious sign and must be reported as soon as possible.

Oedema is swelling due to fluid collecting in the tissues. The skin at the site of the oedema pits on pressure by the fingers, the mark remaining visible for a few seconds.

Behaviour is often an indication of the patient's condition. Irritability and depression may be the result of some physical or mental maladjustment. The over-cheerful patient may also be reacting to some problem, particularly if such behaviour is unusual. Any change in the normal behaviour should be noted and reported.

The temperature

Temperature is measured with a thermometer. There are two scales of temperature, the Fahrenheit scale (F) and the other is the Celsius (or Centigrade) scale (C). These two scales are compared in Fig. 4.1.

The body temperature in health ranges between 36°C and 37.2°C (97°F and 99°F) with an average normal temperature of 36.9°C (98.4°F). It also varies at different times of the day, the evening temperature being about one degree higher than that of the morning.

The clinical thermometer is used for recording body temperature. It is made of glass with a hollow tube running through the centre. At one end is a bulb containing mercury which rises into the centre tube when heated. The mercury will not return to the bulb until the thermometer is shaken, because there is a constriction in the tube which prevents this. Care should be taken when shaking the thermometer that it is held firmly and that it does not come into contact with nearby

Care of the patient 21

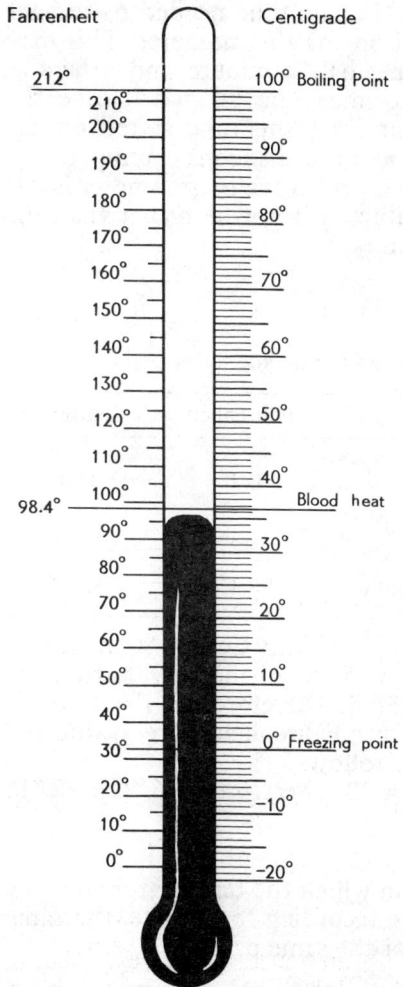

Fig. 4.1 Thermometer showing Fahrenheit and Celsius (Centigrade) degrees.

furniture or it will break.

Degrees of temperature are marked on the clinical thermometer by long black lines with figures varying from 35°C to 43°C or from 95°F to 110°F. Between each of the long lines are four shorter lines, equally spaced so that each degree is divided into five equal parts of 0.2° of temperature. The average normal body temperature is often marked on the thermometer

22　Practical nursing

by an arrow at 36.9°C or 98.4°F. The time needed to register the temperature is also marked on the thermometer. This may vary, some thermometers taking half a minute and others as much as three minutes. Care must be taken to leave the thermometer in position for at least the time stated on the thermometer. If it is removed too soon, an incorrect temperature will be recorded. However long a period the thermometer is left in place, the recorded temperature will not be higher than the body temperature of the patient.

Temperature scales (Table 4.1)

Table 4.1 Comparison of Fahrenheit and Centigrade scales

	Fahrenheit	Centigrade
Boiling point of water at normal atmospheric pressure	212°	100°
Freezing point of water at normal atmospheric pressure	32°	0°
Normal temperature of the human body	98.4°	36.9°

1. To convert Fahrenheit degrees into Celsius (Centigrade) degrees. Subtract 32, multiply by 5 and divide by 9, as follows: 98 - 32 = 66 x 5 = 330 ÷ 9 = 36.6. Therefore 98 °F = 36.6 °C.
2. To convert Celsius degrees into Fahrenheit degrees. Multiply by 9, divide by 5 and add 32, as follows:
36.6 x 9 = 330 ÷ 5 = 66 + 32 = 98. Therefore 36.6 °C = 98 °F.

Taking the temperature
There are four suitable places in which the temperature may be taken, but as the reading varies according to the site, the same place must be used each time for the same patient.

1. The mouth.
2. The axilla. ⎫ The temperature is the same in these
3. The groin.　⎭ positions, being about 0.5°-1° lower than in the mouth.
4. The rectum.　This temperature is about 0.5°- 1° higher than in the mouth.

Taking the temperature in the mouth　The mercury is shaken down to below 35.5°C (96°F) and the thermometer wiped before placing underneath the patient's tongue. The lips should be closed, but not the teeth, and the patient should be told not to talk whilst the thermometer is in place. The thermometer is left in position for the requisite time, then removed and the temperature recorded. The thermometer is shaken so that the mercury is below 35.5°C (96°F) and replaced in antiseptic.

When taking the temperature the patient should be sitting or lying down; it should not be taken immediately after a hot bath, after smoking, or after drinking hot or very cold fluids, because these factors affect the temperature recorded on the thermometer. The temperature should not be taken in the mouth for very young children, unconscious, delirious and irresponsible patients, where there is difficulty in breathing or in diseases of the mouth.

Taking the temperature in the axilla or groin The skin should be dried thoroughly before placing the thermometer in position, and the thermometer must be in contact with the skin on all sides, with no clothing intervening, or it will not register correctly. The arm is drawn across the chest and held in place until the thermometer has registered. The same principles apply where the temperature is taken in the groin. The leg is drawn across the abdomen and held in position for the required time. This is especially important when taking the temperature of a child in the groin.

Taking a temperature in the rectum A special thermometer with a rounded bulb is used, which is kept separate from other thermometers. The bulb is lubricated with Vaseline or liquid paraffin, gently inserted into the rectum for about 2.5 cm (1 in) and held there until the temperature is recorded. This method is used for small children and babies. The child's legs must be firmly and gently controlled by the nurse whilst holding the thermometer in place in the rectum, but if the child is restless, two nurses may be needed. After removal, the thermometer should be washed in warm, soapy water, rinsed and replaced in disinfectant.

Ranges of temperature

	Degrees centigrade
Normal range	36.1 - 37.2
Pyrexia	37.2 - 40.6
Hyperpyrexia	Above 40.6
Hypothermia	Below 35

Temperature charts
A chart is kept for every patient, which enables the medical and senior nursing staff to see at a glance the general condition and

24 Practical nursing

progress of the patient. On this chart are recorded the daily temperature, pulse and respiration rates, and any other information it may be necessary to record, such as the amount of urine passed, the results of urine tests, bowel action, special drugs given, treatments, operations or any other unusual occurrences concerning the patient.

Temperatures are taken every morning and evening, or four-hourly, and are charted accordingly. Special pulse-rate charts are used where the pulse rate is taken every quarter or half hour, as in cases of severe illness or after operation.

Charting must be done neatly and accurately.

Rigor

The sudden onset of severe illness is often marked by a rigor, which occurs in three definite stages.

1. *The cold stage.* The patient complains of feeling very cold and shivers so violently as to shake the bed. The skin may be cold and blue, and the temperature begins to rise.

2. *The hot stage.* The skin becomes hot and dry, the patient complains of thirst and headache, the temperature continues to rise and the pulse is rapid.

3. *The sweating stage.* This follows the hot stage after a varying length of time. There is profuse sweating and the clothing and bedding become damp. The temperature falls and the pulse rate becomes less rapid. The patient is often exhausted after a rigor and needs skilled nursing care.

Treatment of a rigor

The patient must not be left alone until recovery is complete. The temperature is taken in the axilla and recorded every ten to fifteen minutes throughout the duration of the rigor.

Cold stage Extra blankets or electric blankets should be supplied. Hot drinks may be given if the patient is able to control the shivering sufficiently to drink. The time the attack commenced should be noted and reported.

Hot stage Some of the blankets may be removed, but care must be taken that the patient does not become chilled. Cold compresses may be applied to the forehead and a cool drink given. Watch must be kept for the beginning of the third stage.

Third stage During this stage the temperature falls. The patient should be kept warmly covered and perspiration wiped only from the face. No further steps should be taken until sweating has ceased. The patient is then dried thoroughly with warmed towels and the clothing, bedding and pillow-cases changed. The bed should remain screened and the patient left to rest until recovery is complete.

Tepid sponging
This treatment is carried out to reduce an extremely high temperature and to make the patient feel more comfortable. The temperature is taken before, during and after the sponging. It will usually fall about 2°, but should the patient complain of feeling cold or a fall of more than 2° be recorded, the sponging must be stopped, and the patient made comfortable and allowed to rest.

Trolley for tepid sponging
Top shelf
Washing bowl with water at 38°C (100°F).
Jug of cold water, small bowl containing ice.
Cold compress.
Clinical thermometer, bath thermometer.
Face cloth, 5 disposable cloths or sponges. Talcum powder. Hair brush. Bath towels.
Lower shelf.
Clean linen. Clean clothes.
In addition — soiled linen container.

Method Tepid sponging should take about twenty minutes to complete. Close the windows to exclude draught, screen the bed and explain to the patient what is to be done. Bring the trolley to the bedside and place the sponges in tepid water. Take the patient's temperature and record it. Strip the bed, leaving the patient covered with the top sheet.

Apply a cold compress to the forehead and place a sponge, wrung out in tepid water, in each axilla and one in each hand. Sponge and dry the face, then proceed as for a blanket bath (see p. 38), using long, sweeping strokes. Each sponge is used once only then wrung out in the tepid water. As the water becomes warmer, cold water should be added and the temperature checked with the bath thermometer.

When sponging of the upper part of the body has been completed the patient's temperature is taken and again recorded. The sponges are removed from the axillae, cooled in the water and placed, one in each groin, while the lower limbs are being treated. As each part of the body is dealt with it should be covered with the sheet to prevent the patient becoming chilled.

Where the body temperature is very high, towels may not be needed to dry the skin, the heat from the body will evaporate the moisture, thus helping to reduce the temperature.

After sponging is completed, the patient's clothing and the bed linen should be changed with as little disturbance as possible. The temperature is taken and a cool drink given, if allowed, after which the patient should have complete rest.

The pulse

The pulse is an important guide to the condition of the patient. It is the wave of expansion which occurs in an artery as blood is pumped through with each contraction of the ventricles of the heart. The pulse can be felt wherever a superficial artery passes over a bone, as at the wrist or at the temple. Various factors influence the pulse rate, e.g. emotion, exercise, drugs, disease and the position of the patient, who should be sitting or lying down whilst the count is being taken. The average normal pulse rate is seventy-two beats per minute.

Variations in the pulse rate

Table 4.2 Ranges of normal pulse rates at varying stages in life

	Beats per minute
Infancy	140
At 12 months of age	120
Childhood	100-90
Adults	80-60

It will be seen from Table 4.2 that the pulse rate becomes slower with increasing age.

When taking the pulse, the rate, rhythm and volume are noted.

The *rate* is the speed at which the heart is beating.

The *rhythm* is the regularity of the beat and the intervals between the beats, which should be of equal duration.

The *volume* is the strength of the beat and indicates the amount of blood in the artery at each contraction. The strength of the pulse may be described as:

(a) *bounding or full*, where it cannot be obliterated by the fingers;

(b) *thready pulse*, which feels like a thread under the fingers and is easily obliterated by compression;

(c) *imperceptible pulse*, which cannot be felt.

Respiration

Respiration consists of two movements, inspiration or breathing in, and expiration or breathing out. During inspiration the ribs are raised by the intercostal muscles (see p. 155). and the diaphragm is lowered. This enlarges the thoracic cavity and increases the capacity of the lungs. When breathing out, the ribs are lowered and the diaphragm rises to help push out impure air from the lungs. It is during *inspiration* that oxygen from the air is passed through the lungs into the blood stream, and with each *expiration* carbon dioxide from the blood is expelled from the lungs. This process is known as the interchange of gases and is the means of supplying the whole body with the oxygen necessary for life. Any interference with respiration causes the body to be deprived of oxygen and the patient will show signs of distress. Such signs should be noted when counting the respirations. The normal adult rate of respiration ranges from sixteen to twenty-four times per minute, and may be increased by excitement, exertion or disease. Respiration rate should always be taken when the patient is at rest and without his knowledge, to avoid any conscious change in the rate, depth or character of the breathing.

Types of respiration

Dyspnoea is difficult breathing.

Orthopnoea means very difficult breathing.

Sighing or yawning (air hunger) is typical of diabetic coma or haemorrhage.

Stertorous breathing is a noisy, snoring inspiration, often heard in disease or injury of the brain.

Cheyne-Stokes respiration is a characteristic type of breathing which may occur during severe illness or on approaching death. The respirations are at first quiet and almost imperceptible, gradually becoming deeper and louder until stertorous in character, after which they gradually die away until breathing appears to cease for a few seconds. The cycle is then resumed, the respirations again becoming progressively louder.

Faeces

Observations of faeces

Faeces constitute the solid waste matter excreted by the lower colon or bowel. Any abnormalities must be noted and reported

28 Practical nursing

by the nurse. Observations will include:
(a) colour and consistency;
(b) frequency with which stools are passed;
(c) the presence of foreign bodies or parasites.

Colour and consistency
Putty-coloured stools occur where the quantity of bile in the colon is reduced or absent so that fats are not efficiently digested. Bile also acts as a disinfectant and helps to reduce odour, therefore, in the absence of bile, these stools are offensive.

Tarry, shiny, semi-solid stools, known as *melaena*, contain digested blood and are an indication of haemorrhage in the upper part of the alimentary tract. Melaena must be reported to senior nursing staff as soon as seen. It is an extremely serious sign. Black, formed stools may be due to certain drugs, such as those containing iron, and must not be confused with melaena.

Bright red blood indicates bleeding from the rectum or anus.

Green stools from babies may be due to defective feeding or to illness. These stools are very acid and will cause the skin of the legs and buttocks to become sore. The napkins must be changed as soon as soiled and the skin well washed and protected with cream.

Frequency
Infrequent passage of faeces is known as *constipation*, a condition which must be noted and reported by the nurse. Solid waste matter collected in the colon may be the cause of ill health and complications, if allowed to continue. *Diarrhoea* is the frequent passage of watery stools which are difficult for the patient to control. This should not be confused with the action of aperients which may produce frequency, but does not constitute diarrhoea.

Foreign bodies
These may consist of inanimate objects such as needles, pins, coins etc., or of animal parasites such as tape worms, thread worms or round worms.

A *tape worm* has a small head and a body made up of many segments and may grow to a length of many feet. The head remains firmly attached to the mucous membrane lining the intestine and the segments drop off and can be seen as white flecks in the stools. Until the head is dislodged the segments continue to grow. Stools are examined and the segments sent to the pathological laboratory for examination. The nurse is responsible for observation of all stools passed by the patient and for reporting the results.

Thread worms are common, especially in children. They appear as tiny white threads around the anus and in faeces. Reinfection constantly takes place by the child's hands being put into the mouth after being in contact with the worms and their eggs.

Round worms occur as a result of taking impure food or water. These worms resemble earthworms in appearance and inhabit the intestines, causing abdominal discomfort. In small children the effects tend to be more serious and may lead to convulsions.

Any stool having a suspected abnormality should be reported to a trained nurse and saved for inspection. The bedpan should be covered and left in the sluice until the contents have been inspected. Stools from a baby are left in the napkin in a covered receptacle and left in the sluice until inspected. Specimens to be sent to the pathological laboratory should be taken from the bedpan with forceps or wooden spatula, free of toilet paper, and placed in a glass or waxed container, labelled with the name of the patient, the ward, and the date.

Suppositories

Suppositories are cone-shaped preparations containing medicaments.

Reasons for giving suppositories

1. To evacuate the bowel instead of using an enema.
2. To administer a drug, e.g. when it is not possible for it to be taken orally.
3. To relieve local discomfort

Requirements on tray

Prescribed suppository.
Patient's prescription sheet.
Lubricant.
Medical wipes.
Disposable glove.
Disposal bag or pedal bin for soiled articles.

Method

The bed is screened and the procedure explained to the patient. The bed-clothes are folded back and the patient is protected with a small blanket. The patient lies in the left lateral position with the knees well flexed and the buttocks at the edge of the bed. The disposable glove is put on the nurse's right hand and well lubricated, and the suppository inserted through the anal sphincter with the index finger. The medical wipe is used to cleanse the anal area and disposed of with with the polythene glove. The patient is made comfortable and reassured that toilet facilities are available. It is important that the patient understands whether the suppository has been given to assist bowel evacuation or whether it has to be retained.

Enemata

An enema is an injection of fluid into the lower bowel through the rectum. It is never given unless ordered by a doctor.

Reasons for giving enemata

1. To clear the lower bowel of faeces.
2. To relieve abdominal discomfort or distension.
3. For diagnostic purposes.
4. To administer drugs or fluids through the rectum.

The type of evacuant enema now most commonly used is the disposable type. Enemata of this type are commercially made and come packaged ready for administration. The requirements and method of administration are as for giving suppositories, but a bedpan and toilet tissue should be brought to the bedside at the beginning of the procedure in case the patient is unable to retain the fluid. The bed should be protected with disposable, waterproof sheeting.

Soap and water enema

This may occasionally be prescribed. Normally, 600-900 ml are given to an adult and a maximum of 30 ml per year of life to a child.

Enema trolley

Measuring jug containing solution — 40 ml of green, soft soap to 600 ml of water.
Lotion, thermometer.

Funnel, length of tubing, connection spring clip.
Rectal catheter.
Lubricant.
Medical wipes.
Waterproof sheeting for bed or trolley.
Plastic apron for the nurse.
Receptacle for soiled articles.
Bedpan and toilet tissue.

Method

The patient is prepared as for giving a suppository and the bed is well protected with waterproof sheeting.

The catheter is well lubricated and attached to the connection and tubing. All air is expelled from the apparatus by running through a little of the fluid and fastening the spring clip. The catheter is inserted for about 10 cm and the clip on the tubing released to allow the fluid to flow slowly into the rectum. During this stage the patient should be persuaded to breathe through the mouth; this helps to reduce muscular tension. When all the fluid has been injected the catheter is carefully withdrawn, disconnected from the rest of the apparatus and placed in the receiver provided. The patient should be encouraged to retain the enema for a few minutes to ensure a satisfactory result. A pad of cotton wool placed against the anus will give confidence and assist the retention of the fluid.

A bedpan is given and the patient well supported with pillows.

Before leaving the bedside, the nurse must make quite certain that the patient is feeling well and that there is no danger of fainting or falling out of bed. Occasionally, collapse or shock may follow the administration of an enema and watch should be kept for any signs of nausea or malaise. The result of the enema must not be thrown away until it has been reported and instructions received as to its disposal.

If the enema is not returned, this fact must also be reported. The fluid must be syphoned back with a tube and funnel into a pail.

On completion of the procedure, the catheter is disposed of and the remainder of the equipment washed in hot, soapy water.

Special enemata

Olive oil enema is given to soften hard or impacted faeces or after operations on the rectum to avoid painful evacuation of waste matter: 175-275 ml (6-10 oz) of warmed olive oil is injected slowly into the rectum through a tube and funnel. The apparatus should be immersed in hot water before use to help the olive oil to run in more easily. The oil should be warmed to a temperature of 37.2 °C (99 °F) by standing the container in a bowl of hot water. The enema should be retained for about half an hour and may be followed by a soap-and-water enema to assist in clearing the lower colon.

Rectal washout

This procedure is carried out when it is necessary to clear the rectum and lower colon of faecal matter, as before the administration of a barium enema in the x-ray department or before examination or operation via the rectum.

Requirements for a rectal washout

The requirements will be the same as for an enema (see p. 30), except that water or saline is used. In addition, a waterproof sheet for the floor and a pail with a lid will be required.

Method

Explain the procedure to the patient, screen the bed and prepare the patient as for the enema (see p. 30). Place the waterproof floor sheet and pail in position near the bed. Expel the air from the apparatus by running a little water through and fasten the clip. Lubricate and insert the catheter into the rectum. Pour a little water into the funnel, release the clip and pour slowly until about 600 ml (or 1 pint) have been used, then invert the funnel over the bucket and allow the fluid to run back. Repeat this process until the water returns clear. The amount of water used and the amount returned must be measured to ensure that none has been retained.

Treatment of flatus

Flatus is an accumulation of gases in the intestine, causing abdominal distension. A flatus or rectal tube is passed to relieve this distension and to make the patient more comfortable.

Requirements

A bowl of warm water and disinfectant.
A bowl containing the rectal tube, connection and rubber tubing.
Lubricant.
Medical swabs.
Waterproof sheeting to protect mattress.
Receiver or pedal bin for soiled articles.

Method
Explain the procedure to the patient and screen the bed. Turn the patient into the left lateral position with the waterproof and small sheets under the buttocks. Place the bowl of water and disinfectant on a chair by the bed. Lubricate the rectal rube and insert gently into the rectum, leaving the open end of the tube under the water in the bowl. Leave in position for ten to fifteen minutes. When flatus is expelled, bubbles will appear in the water. The patient should not be left until the treatment is completed because the amount of flatus passed must be noted and reported. After the requisite time, remove the flatus tube and make the patient comfortable.

Tray for rectal examination

A selection of disposable gloves.
Fingercots.
Tube KY Jelly.
Disposal bags.
Medical wipes.
Disposable towel to protect the bed.

Method
The bladder and rectum should be emptied before rectal examination. The skin round the anus should be very clean. The patient should be placed in the left lateral position and not exposed unduly.

Colostomy washout

A colostomy is an artificial opening made into the colon, where there is disease or obstruction of any part of the large intestine or rectum; it may be temporary or permanent. A loop of the colon is brought to the surface of the abdomen above the site of the obstruction, and an opening made, through which faecal matter is drained. Two channels open into this loop, the *active* opening, leading away from the diseased area and through which waste matter passes, and the *non-active* opening leading towards the affected part.

Good nursing of these cases is most important to prevent the skin of the abdomen becoming sore. Patients with a colostomy are often miserable and depressed on realizing its implications; to a sensitive person it is unpleasant and distressing. The nurse can do much to lessen the distress by explaining that the action of the colostomy will become more regular as time passes. Many hospitals now employ stoma therapists who are expert in fitting the many appliances now available and in giving guidance and support to the patient. National agencies such as the Ileostomy Association can give valuable help to such patients.

Colostomy washout

The requirements and method are as for rectal washout (see p. 32), with the addition of fresh appliance and any necessary barrier creams. The patient should be turned towards the affected side.

Caecostomy

A caecostomy is an artificial opening into the caecum (the first part of the large intestine); it is usually a temporary measure. Liquid faecal matter is discharged from the small intestine and is extremely irritating to the skin of the abdomen, which may become sore in consequence.

Frequent attention is essential in order to keep the skin in good condition.

Unlike a colostomy, the action of a caecostomy cannot at any time be controlled. A special belt fitted with a plastic bag is worn.

5
The skin

The formation and function of the skin

The skin consists of two layers, the outer layer or *epidermis* and the *dermis* or true skin. The epidermis forms the covering for the whole body and is thickest on the hands and feet. It is made up of several layers of cells which are continually rubbed off and replaced from underneath. The nails are formed by certain of the flattened, epithelial cells being changed into hard, horny plates.

The *epidermis* contains no blood vessels or glands and few nerves, but it contains pigment which gives colour to the skin. Its surface is covered with minute openings, called pores, through which sweat is excreted from the sweat glands in the dermis.

The *dermis*, or true skin, lies under the epidermis and contains the following structures by which the skin functions.
1. Blood and lymphatic vessels.
2. Nerves of touch.
3. Sebaceous glands which secrete an oily substance called sebum.
4. Sweat glands which open to the surface of the epidermis.
5. Hair follices from which the hairs grow (Fig. 5.1).

Functions of the skin
1. To protect the body from injury and the entrance of harmful bacteria.
2. To excrete waste matter as sweat, i.e. water and salts.
3. To regulate the body temperature by the action of the sweat glands and by radiation.
4. To produce vitamin D by the action of ultraviolet light.
5. It is the organ of touch and gives sensations of heat, cold or pain.

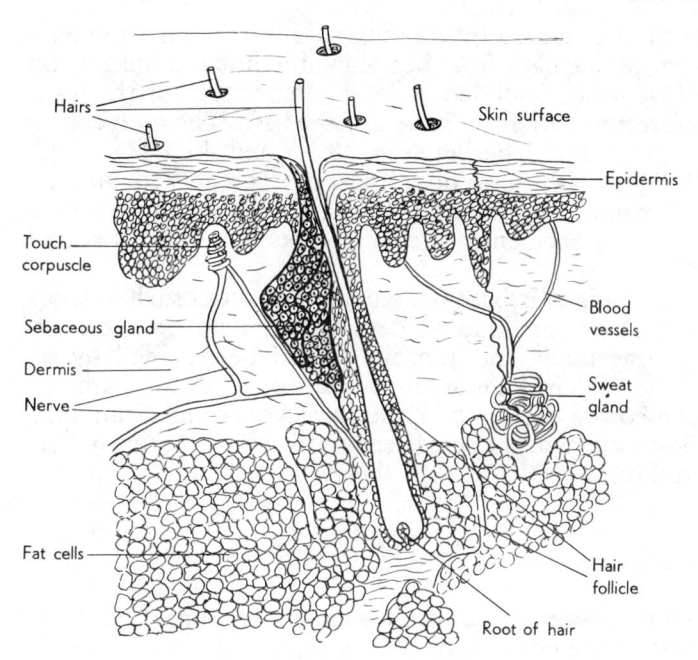

Fig. 5.1 Formation of the skin.

Care of the skin

The utmost care must be taken of the skin if it is to function efficiently. In sickness it is doubly important that the proper working of the skin structures is ensured, and that waste matter is not allowed to accumulate.

The patient should be washed twice a day and, when confined to bed, blanket bathed every day. Those who get up can use the bathroom daily. All patients are bathed on admission, unless there are exceptional circumstances which make a bath impossible. For patients admitted from the waiting list the bath may be deferred until bedtime at the discretion of the nurse in charge.

Bathing in the bathroom

The nurse is responsible for the preparation of the bath for the patient. All equipment required should be collected and taken into the bathroom, the windows closed and a screen placed in front of the door to ensure privacy.

The bath is prepared by running cold water first to prevent the bottom of the bath from becoming too hot and burning the patient. Hot water is added and the temperature of the water taken before the patient commences the bath. The temperature of a hot bath should be between 38 °C and 43.5 °C (100 °-110 °F). The bathroom door must not be locked and the patient must not be left alone in the bathroom for any length of time, in case of accident or collapse. The nurse should remain within call.

While the patient is bathing, any abnormalities such as spots, wounds, scars or any kind of deformity should be noted and reported. Fingernails and toenails should be trimmed by the nurse, if the patient cannot do this alone. After the bath, the patient is escorted back to bed, the bath cleaned and disinfected, the windows opened, the screen removed and the bathroom left clean and tidy.

Blanket bathing

Requirements (assembled on trolley and locker top)
  Bowl with hand hot water.
  Soap.
  Two face cloths.
  One bath towel.
  One face towel.
  Talcum powder.
  Toothbrush/paste/mug/receiver.
  Nailbrush ⎫
  Nail scissors ⎬ as necessary.
  Hair brush. ⎭
  Bathing blanket (many hospitals now use the top sheet for this purpose and change it at the end of the bath).
  Clean clothing.
  Clean bed linen.
  Receptacle for soiled linen.

Method
The patient is told what is to be done and the trolley taken to the bedside. The windows are closed and the bed screened. The bed-clothes are removed as far as the top sheet and either this is left covering the patient and changed at the end of the procedure, or a bathing blanket is put in position and the sheet removed from under it.

The washing should be carried out quickly and thoroughly, without undue exposure or chilling of the patient. The face, arms, chest, abdomen, legs and back are taken in that order, each part being washed, thoroughly dried, lightly powdered and covered, before proceeding with the next section. Where possible, the patient may prefer to wash the groin and genitals, in which case the nurse must see that everything needed is within easy reach.

Where two folds of the skin are in contact, special care must be taken to ensure complete dryness.

All pressure areas should be treated during the bath. The skin over bony prominences such as the shoulders, hips, elbows or heels should be well massaged with soap and water, then dried and dusted with powder. Fingernails and toenails should be trimmed.

When the bath is completed the patient is dressed in a clean, warmed bedgown or pyjamas and left warm and comfortable in a freshly made bed. Following the blanket bath, the mouth and hair should receive attention.

Care of the mouth

The mouth is lined with mucous membrane which secretes mucus to keep the inside of the mouth and the lips moist. In very ill patients the mucous membrane becomes dry and may crack giving rise to sores inside the mouth known as *sordes*. Cracks and sores outside the mouth are called *herpes*. Where the patient is unable to clean the teeth, a mouth tray is needed, especially for the following.

    Severely ill patients.
    Patients with pyrexia or hyperpyrexia.
    Paralysed or otherwise helpless patients.
    Patients suffering from diseases of the mouth.
    Those taking no food or fluid by mouth.

Complications of a neglected mouth include sordes, herpes, nausea, refusal of food, inflammation of the mucous membrane of the stomach, sepsis of the respiratory tract, tonsillitis and swollen glands.

The mouth tray
    One small disposable towel.
    Medical wipes.
    Sodium bicarbonate, 1 teaspoonful to 540 ml of water.
    Glycerin of thymol, 1 tablet to a tumblerful of water.

Glycerin to moisten mouth.
Vaseline for lips to prevent drying and cracking.
Cotton-wool balls or dental rolls.
One pair of artery forceps.
One pair of dissecting forceps.
Wooden applicators
Paper bag or other receptacle for soiled articles.

Method
The towel is placed under the patient's chin. Dentures, if any, must be removed and, using the patient's toothbrush, should be scrubbed and rinsed under running water and placed in a denture box with water.

Every part of the inside of the mouth is swabbed with bicarbonate of soda, using dental rolls or cotton-wool balls held firmly with the artery forceps. These are removed when soiled with the dissecting forceps and dropped into the paper bag. This procedure is repeated with the Glycothymoline, followed by the glycerine and borax. The wooden applicators with tiny wool swabs attached are used to clean between the teeth. After use they are broken and placed with the soiled swabs in a receiver. Where there are sores round the mouth, cream or ointment should be applied with a clean swab.

Care of the scalp and hair

The hair and scalp of all new admissions is examined for infestation by pediculi (head lice). The general care of the hair includes brushing and combing twice a day. If the patient is unable to do this, the nurse should brush and comb the hair regularly to keep it free from knots and dust, to promote circulation of blood through the scalp and to make the patient feel comfortable. If the hair is long, it is most manageable if dressed in two plaits, one on each side of the head. In cases of infestation a head tray will be required to cleanse the hair.

Head tray

Gown and head covering for the nurse.
Bowl of wool swabs.
Bowl of disinfectant containing a small tooth comb.
Gallipot containing Prioderm, Lorexane or Suleo.
Receiver of disinfectant for soiled swabs.

Receiver with brush and comb.
Waterproof cape.

Method
The hair is combed to remove knots, then treated, one lock at a time. The fine-tooth comb is dipped into disinfectant and drawn through the lock of hair from the scalp downwards. After each combing the tooth comb is rinsed in the disinfectant. This process is repeated until the whole head has been dealt with. Each lock of hair should then be swabbed with one of the special preparations, using each swab once only, until all the hair has been treated.

Washing the hair in bed
The skin of the scalp must be kept clean for the comfort of the patient. Where hair cannot be washed in the bathroom it must be done in bed. The head of the bed, where possible, is removed and the mattress pulled down so that the bowl of water rests on the spring, or the bowl may be placed on a chair near the top of the bed. The mattress is protected with waterproof sheeting, which should reach from under the patient's shoulders into a pail placed on the floor, forming a channel by which the water drains into the bucket. A waterproof cape and towel are placed round the patient's shoulders and a waterproof covered pillow under the hair.

The hair is shampooed and rinsed twice, making sure that all soap is removed. Water is squeezed from the hair and a towel wrapped around the head until the bowl, waterproof sheets, towels and shoulder cape are removed, the mattress and pillows replaced and the patient made comfortable. The hair may then be spread over the mackintosh-protected pillow, covered with a towel and dried with warm towels or a hair drier. When dry, the hair is arranged as attractively as possible.

If the head of the bed cannot be removed, the patient may be placed in the left lateral position or may lie across the bed with the feet resting on a chair. Care must be taken that the patient is well covered with blankets.

Trolley for washing the hair in bed
  Shampoo.
  Brush and comb.
  Small jug for rinsing.
  Bowl of warm water.

Face cloth.
Shoulder cape.
Bath towel.
Hair dryer.
Plastic apron for nurse.
Waterproof sheeting to protect bedding.

Pressure sores

Patients confined to bed for any length of time are liable to develop bed-sores and it is the aim of the nurse to prevent this wherever possible. Bed-sores may be the result of inferior nursing care, because in most cases they can be prevented. A bed-sore is an ulcer which may form over bony prominences or where two surfaces of skin are in close contact, as in the axillae or under the breasts, especially in very fat people. The first sign is redness of the skin, soreness and discomfort, which, if neglected, will result in cracks leading to an open wound. Because of the rapidity with which a bed-sore may develop, frequent attention must be given to all areas of the body which may become affected.

Causes of bed-sores

1. Pressure: from lying or sitting too long in one position.
2. Friction: from creased or patched sheets and from crumbs in the bed, or from carelessly handled bedpans.
3. Moisture: as during incontinence or excessive sweating.
4. Irritation: caused by skin rashes or excreta.
5. Injury: cracks or abrasions caused by careless handling of the patient, by wristwatches, rings, or long fingernails of a nurse.
Types of patients liable to bed-sores are helpless, unconscious, paralysed, incontinent, extremely fat or thin patients and those who are severely ill.

Common pressure areas

These are at the back of the head, shoulder-blades and points of the shoulders, elbows, vertebrae, hips and sacral areas, knees, toes, heels and ankles (Fig. 5.2).

In the prevention of pressure sores the object is to stimulate the circulation of blood to the part in order to keep the tissues nourished. This is assisted by:

1. changing the position of the patient at frequent intervals;

The skin 43

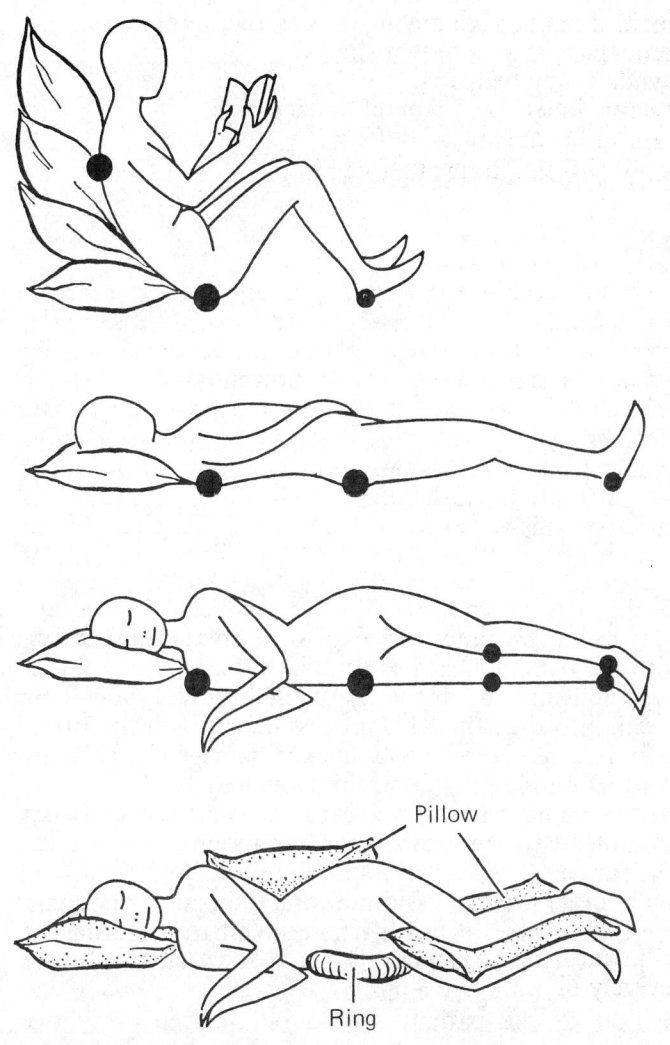

Fig. 5.2 Pressure areas. Bottom figure shows how to place pillows to relieve pressure. (From Darwin *et al.*, (19). *Bedside Nursing: An Introduction*. Heinemann, London.)

2. routine treatment twice a day and more often where necessary;
3. the use of such equipment as ripple beds, air beds, rings or ring pads to relieve pressure;

44 Practical nursing

    4. careful bed-making, removing creases and crumbs from the bed and frequent changing of wet sheets;
    5. care when giving bedpans;
    6. good nourishment and general nursing care.

Routine treatment to prevent bed-sores

Requirements
    Wash bowl with warm water.
    Soap.
    Talcum powder.
    Towel.
    Preferred barrier cream.
    Clean linen.
    Clean clothing.
    Incontinence pads, if necessary.
    Receptacle for soiled pads.
    Receptacle for soiled linen.

Method
Explain to the patient what is to be done. Screen the bed and close windows. Expose only the area to be treated, protecting the bed with the patient's bath towel. Wash the area gently with soap and water. Rinse and dry well, dust lightly with powder or massage cream into the skin. This process must be gently carried out; hard rubbing is dangerous and may damage the skin. All pressure areas should be treated in the same manner.

Straighten or replace the drawsheet and leave the patient dry and comfortable. The water should be hot and must be changed for each patient.

Silicone or other barrier creams protect the skin and assist healing where the skin is broken. Where such barrier creams are in use, the pressure areas need not be washed more than once a day, unless there is soiling by excreta.

The position of the patient should be changed every two hours. This relieves pressure, allowing the blood to flow more freely over the affected areas. This is an extremely important point in the prevention and treatment of pressure sores.

Profuse sweating

This is an important sign and should never be overlooked. It may indicate the onset of severe illness or coma. Persistent profuse sweating will result in loss of body fluids and salts without which the body cannot function efficiently. These fluids must therefore be replaced by giving the patient extra fluids by mouth, nasogastrically or intravenously. The skin must be sponged twice daily and watch kept for any sign of chafing or bed-sores.

Diseases of the skin

These may be inherited or acquired and affect any of the structures in the dermis or epidermis. Such diseases include:
1. those affecting the sebaceous or sweat glands;
2. those affecting the growth of epithelial cells;
3. inflammatory conditions;
4. disorders of the nerves of the skin;
5. attacks by animal or vegetable parasites.

The care of patients suffering from skin diseases is of great importance because these diseases have an influence on mental as well as physical health. Changes that take place in the skin are usually unpleasant and sometimes alter the appearance. The patient is often acutely aware of this and may be highly sensitive to the reaction of other people. Patients suffering from skin lesions must not be made to feel embarrassed in any way. They should be treated with the utmost kindness and consideration and at no time should reference be made to the appearance of the skin.

General symptoms include tingling, burning, soreness, irritation and, more rarely, pain. Treatment varies according to the cause and type of the disease.

The *most common lesions* seen in disorders of the skin are as follows.

Macule   A slight area of discolouration not raised above the level of the surrounding skin.

Vesicle or *blister*   A small sac of clear fluid.

Pustule   A similar sac containing pus.

Papule or *pimple*   A raised, solid spot.

Crusts   Appear when a vesicle or pustule perforates and the fluid dries on the skin.

Scales   Dried epithelial cells which flake off the surface of the skin.

Weals   Raised white swellings with bright red edges.

Purpura   Small patches of haemorrhage appearing underneath the skin.

Erythema   A condition in which irregular areas of skin becomes red and irritable.

Common disorders of the skin

Acne

Acne is a chronic condition which affects the sebaceous glands and hair follicles causing the formation of pustules and papules on the surface of the skin. It occurs in young people between 14 and 20 years of age, but usually disappears spontaneously within two years of onset.

Boils

Boils are the result of infection of hair follicles by staphylococci resulting in the formation of pus. A collection of boils in one area forms a large, open, septic wound known as a *carbuncle*.

Corns and callouses

Corns and callouses are due to an overgrowth and thickening of the epidermis, causing pressure on underlying nerve endings and producing pain.

Dermatitis

Dermatitis is a condition due to contact with some irrritating agent such as flour, oil, wood, fur or some species of plant life and some synthetic materials. Treatment varies according to the cause of irritation.

Eczema

Eczema is inflammation of the skin caused by an irritant or by bacterial invasion. Some types of eczema are associated with asthma. In all cases the use of soap and water on the skin is to be avoided; oily preparations should be used for cleansing.

Infantile eczema

Infantile eczema usually affects children under the age of 2 years. To prevent the child from scratching, the arms are placed in cardboard splints until the irritation and inflammation have subsided.

Erysipelas

Erysipelas is caused by infection by streptococci. It appears as a raised red area on the surface of the skin, accompanied by pain. It is usually to be seen on the face, but may occur around surgical wounds as a result of cross infection. The germs are present in skin lesions.

Herpes zoster

Herpes zoster, or shingles, is a virus infection of nerve cells in the skin causing vesicles to appear, accompanied by severe pain and malaise. These vesicles are distributed along the course of a nerve, commonly on the face and over the forehead or around the body, in the region of the ribs.

Impetigo

Impetigo is an infection of the skin by staphylococci or streptococci. Vesicles and pustules form on the skin and burst. The fluid dries forming crusts, usually on the face. The disease is commonly found in children of all ages. It is extremely infectious and is passed from person to person. The crusts must be removed by bathing or with a starch poultice before being treated with antibiotic cream. Small children should have the arms splinted to prevent them from touching the infected sores. All toys and equipment must be kept away from other people.

Psoriasis

Psoriasis is a chronic disease of unknown origin, but appears to be aggravated by emotional disturbances. It is marked by the appearance of dry, silvery scales forming patches on the skin, although rarely on the face.

Scabies

Scabies is an irritating condition caused by a parasite known commonly as the itch mite. The female insect burrows under the soft skin between the fingers, at the wrists, behind the knees and on the inside aspect of the elbows where it lays its eggs. The eggs hatch and reinfect the skin or clothing. Scabies causes severe itching, especially at night. Scratching may result in secondary infection of the skin by introduction of dirt into the

48 Practical nursing

lesions. The infection can be passed from one person to another by direct contact.

Treatment

Treatment consists of daily bathing in hot soapy water, scrubbing the infected areas to open the burrows made by the itch mite. A lotion such as Quellada is then applied to the entire skin surface, paying special attention to the affected areas. This treatment is repeated in two days and where the itch persists a third treatment may be carried out if necessary. All members of the family should be treated.

Seborrhoea

Seborrhoea is due to excessive secretion by the sebaceous glands in the dermis. Sebum collects on the surface of the skin and, together with dirt and dust, forms crusts. This condition is often seen on the scalp, especially in the young. Where possible the crusts are removed with oily applications and the skin kept as clean as possible.

Sebaceous cysts

Sebaceous cysts are formed by a collection of sebum enclosed in a small sac from which it cannot escape, and eventually appears on the surface as a swelling. Where these cysts cause distress or discomfort they are removed surgically.

Tinea (ringworm)

Tinea or ringworm is due to a vegetable parasite or fungus which may affect the hair, skin or nails.

Ringworm of the skin is commonly found on the feet, causing the skin between the toes to become white, moist and irritable. Infection may be spread by contact with wet floors in such public places as swimming pools or baths. The fungi may be carried on clothing, so socks or stockings should be washed and changed every day. The skin should be washed daily and dressed as ordered.

Ringworm of the scalp is usually seen in children. The fungi attacks the hairs causing them to break off and fall out until the area becomes bald. X-ray treatment may be ordered to clear the scalp of infected hair. Clothing should be changed daily and everything used by the patient should be disinfected thoroughly after use.

Starch poultice

This may be used for the removal of crusts in such skin diseases as impetigo. It is applied when almost cold and of a jelly-like consistency and is left in place for six to twelve hours.

Requirements

    About 20 ml (1½ tablespoonful) of powdered starch.
    300 ml (½ pint) of boiling water.
    Poultice board and spatula, old linen.
    Mixing bowl and jug, a piece of washed muslin to cover the poultice.
    Receiver for used swabs.
    Warm olive oil for removing the old poultice, dressing forceps and swabs in a bowl; bandages.

Method

The starch is mixed with a little cold water to a thick cream. Boiling water is added slowly until the starch becomes a thick, blue, clear jelly. When cold the jelly is spread about 1.25 cm (0.5 in) thick on old linen, and covered with the muslin. The poultice is covered and bandaged firmly in position.
    When taking off the poultice, any loosely adhering crusts should be gently removed with dissecting forceps, swabs and warm olive oil, and a fresh dressing applied as ordered.

6

The respiratory system

In order to maintain good health, oxygen must be supplied to the tissues and waste matter, in the form of carbon dioxide and water vapour, excreted. The replacement of carbon dioxide with oxygen in the lungs during breathing is spoken of as the interchange of gases.

The respiratory system consists of the nose, the larynx or voice box, the trachea or windpipe, the bronchi and bronchioles and the lungs.

The nose

The nose is lined with mucous membrane, rich in blood vessels, which serves to warm and moisten the air as it enters the nostrils. Dust is filtered out by short, coarse hairs in the lower part of the nose and by ciliated epithelium in the upper nasal passages (see. p. 151).

The nasopharynx

The nasopharynx lies behind the posterior nasal cavities or nostrils. At each side of the nasopharynx are the openings of the Eustachian tubes which lead into the middle ears. On the posterior wall is a collection of lymphoid tissue which, when enlarged, is commonly referred to as adenoids (see p. 96).

The larynx

The larynx (Fig. 6.1) is situated in front of the neck above the trachea. It is made up of several cartilages, the chief of which are the *thyroid* cartilage supporting the thyroid gland and the *epiglottis,* a leaf-shaped cartilage which closes down over the larynx during swallowing to prevent food or drink from entering the trachea and causing choking or asphyxiation. The larynx contains the vocal cords which produce sound as air passes over them.

The respiratory system 51

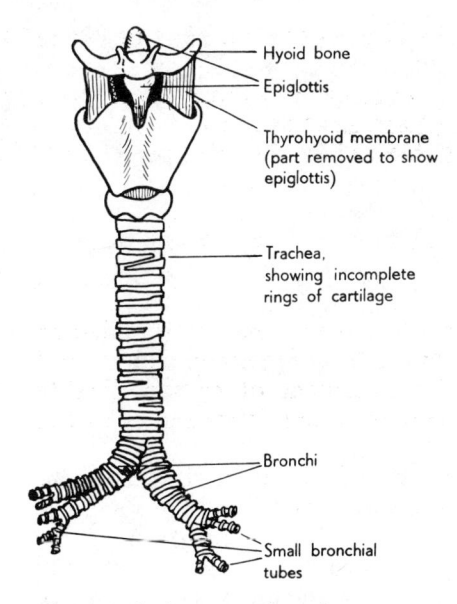

Fig. 6.1 The larynx and trachea.

The trachea
The trachea (Fig. 6.1) is a tube, about 11 cm (4.5 in) long, made up of incomplete rings of cartilage that prevent it collapsing. The gap in each ring lies at the back of the trachea against the oesophagus; this allows the wall of the trachea to give slightly during the action of swallowing. The trachea is lined with ciliated epithelium which helps to keep it free of irritating substances.

The bronchi
At the level of the fifth thoracic vertebra the trachea divides into the right and left bronchi. These penetrate into the right and left lungs, then divide into still smaller branchs called bronchioles. Each bronchiole ends in a small cluster of air sacs or alveoli.

The lungs
The lungs are two cone-shaped organs, situated one on each side of the thorax (Fig. 6.2). The base of each lung rests on the

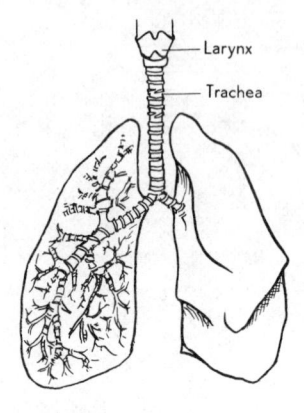

Fig. 6.2 The lungs.

diaphragm; the apex stands about 2.5 cm (1 in) above the clavicle. The right lung is divided into three lobes and the left lung into two lobes. The substance of the lungs is composed of spongy tissue made up of clusters of air sacs. The walls of each air sac consist of a single layer of cells surrounded by capillaries, so that the entire surface of the lungs is covered with a network of tiny blood vessels. Through the walls of the air sacs and capillaries, the interchange of gases takes place. Oxygen passes from the air sacs into the blood and carbon dioxide and moisture is passed from the bloodstream into the air sacs to be excreted during respiration.

The pleura
The pleura is a double layer of serous membrane, the outer layer lining the chest wall and the other turned back to cover the lungs. Between these two layers pleural fluid is secreted, which acts as a lubricant, preventing the two layers of the pleura from sticking together and enabling the lungs to move freely without friction.

Common respiratory diseases

Respiratory diseases are those affecting any part of the respiratory system. Common symptoms are cough, sputum, pain in the chest, dyspnoea (difficult breathing), cyanosis (blueness of the face), and in severe cases there may be haemoptysis (bleeding from the lungs).

The respiratory system

Coryza

Coryza is the technical term for a common cold, for which there is, as yet, no known cure. The chief symptom is rhinitis, or inflammation of the mucous membrane lining the nose, resulting in excessive outpouring of fluid from the nasal passages.

Laryngitis

Laryngitis is inflammation of the larynx and vocal cords, resulting in loss of voice. *Acute laryngitis* may be due to the common cold or to some infectious disease. *Chronic laryngitis* may be caused by overstrain of the vocal cords by too much singing or talking, or to disease of the larynx. The treatment varies according to the cause of the inflammation.

Tracheitis

Tracheitis is inflammation of the trachea and is usually a complication of the common cold or of infectious disease such as measles or diphtheria.

Pharyngitis

Pharyngitis is inflammation of the soft palate or pharynx. It is a painful, sore condition often associated with coryza.

Moist inhalations, e.g. friar's balsam, are usually ordered in the treatment of the above conditions.

Bronchitis

Bronchitis is inflammation of the bronchial tubes and may be acute or chronic. *Acute bronchitis* often occurs in young children and may be a complication of teething in the very young or of infectious diseases. It may also occur in the elderly patients and is characterized by persistent cough, white frothy sputum, dyspnoea and a tight feeling in the chest which causes distress. The nursing care of such cases includes warmth, rest in bed in the upright position, a light, nourishing diet, with plenty of fluids, fresh air without draughts, constant attention to the pressure areas, especially of elderly patients, and moist inhalations as ordered. *Chronic bronchitis* recurs each winter particularly amongst elderly people. There is persistent cough with expectoration of sputum.

Emphysema

Emphysema may arise as a result of violent coughing over a long period in which some of the air sacs become strained and distended. Air is trapped in the lung instead of being exhaled and the function of the lung is impaired.

Pneumonia

Pneumonia is caused by the invasion of various micro-organisms resulting in inflammation and congestion of air sacs of the lungs. There are three main types, namely lobar pneumonia, bronchopneumonia and hypostatic pneumonia.

Lobar pneumonia In lobar pneumonia one or more whole lobes of one or both lungs may be affected. The onset is sudden, with pyrexia, rigor, pain in the chest, herpes (sores round the mouth), short, dry cough and dyspnoea. In some cases the pleura covering the affected lobe may become inflamed, giving rise to pleurisy.

Empyema Empyema may be a complication of lobar pneumonia in which pus forms in the pleural cavity or between the lobes of the lungs. This condition is usually treated surgically and the pus drained from the lung.

Hypostatic pneumonia Hypostatic pneumonia is the result of faulty circulation of blood in the lungs and may be due to heart failure or to enforced immobility, as when elderly patients have to remain in bed in the recumbent position for any length of time. Fluid collects at the base of the lungs, causing congestion of the air sacs. Prevention of this condition is most important. The patient should be nursed in the upright position where possible and should be moved frequently in bed. This applies particularly to old people who are encouraged to sit out of bed as soon as their condition permits.

Bronchopneumonia Scattered areas of inflammation occur over the lungs, affecting some of the tiny bronchioles and the air sacs to which they are connected. It may be a complication of bronchitis or of some other disease and often affects children or elderly people.

Nursing care of pneumonia
The patient is on complete bed rest in the upright position, well supported with pillows. This position allows the lungs greater freedom of movement and assists breathing. Care should be taken that the patient does not slip down the bed. A foot board, sand bags or a pillow placed at the feet will help maintain the

upright position. Clothing should be loose and warm and should fasten at the back so that it does not constrict the patient in any way. This also enables any nursing procedure or examination to be carried out with less exhaustion for the patient. Constant attention to the pressure areas must be stressed because these patients quickly develop bed-sores. The diet should be light and nourishing with plenty of fluids. Where there is any degree of exhaustion the patient should be fed by the nurse (see p. 102). Moist inhalations may be ordered and kaolin poultices may be applied to the chest for the relief of pain (see p. 75). Oxygen should be readily available in case of respiratory failure. A four-hourly temperature, pulse and respiration chart must be kept, also a fluid intake and output chart (see p. 83).

Pleurisy

Pleurisy is inflammation of the pleura. There are two types, dry pleurisy and pleurisy with effusion.

Dry pleurisy   Dry pleurisy occurs as a result of the two layers of the pleura becoming inflamed, dry and adherent, causing acute pain with each respiration.

Pleural effusion   Pleural effusion is an increase of the pleural fluid between the layers of the pleura causing pressure on the lungs and giving rise to difficult breathing (dyspnoea). Where the pressure becomes too great the fluid may be withdrawn by aspiration for the relief of pain and discomfort. Empyema may be a complication of pleurisy (see p. 54).

Nursing care of pleurisy

Nursing care of pleurisy is as for pneumonia. Complete bed rest is essential, with extra warmth where necessary and regular treatment of all pressure areas. A patient suffering from pleurisy will usually lie on the affected side in an effort to obliterate the pain. A pillow should be placed along the back on the unaffected side to provide extra support. A four-hourly pulse and respiration chart should be kept, also an intake and output chart. Moist inhalations may be ordered and hot applications applied to the affected side to relieve pain.

Bronchial asthma

Bronchial asthma is a common ailment, usually due to an allergy. A spasm of the bronchus is caused by some irritating substance resulting in dyspnoea, which may last from a few minutes to several days. Treatment varies according to the severity of an attack. Inhalations are often found to be helpful and are given as ordered.

Bronchiectasis

Bronchiectasis is usually secondary to some lung diseases. The bronchi become dilated, forming cavities in the lung. From these cavities the secreted mucus is unable to escape and remains in the lung where it becomes purulent and extremely unpleasant to the patient. Periodic postural drainage is employed in an effort to drain the lung of the accumulated pus and mucus. The patient is placed in the prone position, face downwards, with the foot of the bed raised, and is encouraged to expectorate as much sputum as possible by coughing. Inhalations may be given to assist this process.

Inhalations

Inhalations may be moist or dry and are commonly used in the treatment of respiratory diseases, but are also employed to introduce drugs which act on other systems of the body.

Reasons for giving inhalations

1. To relieve spasm of the bronchial tubes, as in asthma.
2. For inflammation of the upper respiratory passages, e.g. laryngitis or tracheitis.
3. For introducing drugs into the body.

Nelson's inhaler
This is a special earthenware inhaler with two spouts which must face in opposite directions when given to a patient. One is the air inlet and is part of the bowl of the inhaler, the other is a glass spout fixed into the cork through which the steam is inhaled into the mouth.

Requirements for inhalation tray

Nelson's inhaler, standing in a bowl to prevent it from tipping over.

Cover for the inhaler to prevent the patient from being burned.

Gauze swab to cover the mouthpiece and a strip of plaster to fasten it.

Medicine measure or teaspoon in which to measure the drug to be used. This may be Compound Tincture of Benzoin or Menthol crystals.

Sputum carton.

Medical wipes.

Method

Pour boiling water into the inhaler up to the level of the lower spout. Measure the drug as ordered, usually 4 ml of tincture of benzoin to 600 ml of water, and add to the boiling water. Replace the cork and cover the glass mouthpiece with the gauze. Place the inhaler in the cover, tie securely and place in the bowl on the tray, which should be put on a bed-table in front and within easy reach of the patient.

The patient should be sitting upright, well supported with pillows and with a small blanket round the shoulders. Close the windows where necessary. Explain to the patient what is required, i.e. to breathe the vapour through the glass mouthpiece into the mouth and out through the nose and to take care that the inhaler is not tipped towards the chest. The air inlet must not be blocked. If the patient is seriously ill, helpless, very young or aged, the nurse must stay at the bedside during the treatment. After use the mouthpiece must be washed and sterilized.

Administration of oxygen

Oxygen is administered when the patient is unable to obtain sufficient oxygen from the air by natural means, as a result of cardiac, respiratory or blood diseases or of poisoning by gas, when respiration becomes dangerously difficult. Oxygen is supplied in cylinders, which are black with white tops, fitted with a spanner by which the gas may be turned on, and a fine adjustment valve by which the flow is controlled. A flowmeter, marked in litres, is fitted, and indicates the rate of flow of oxygen to the patient, usually from 4 to 6 litres per minute. No spark or flame should be allowed near the cylinder. Because of the danger of explosion or fire, no smoking is allowed near oxygen cylinders or tents. Cylinders should be opened outside the ward where possible and always away from the bedside before the connection is made to the patient. Many hospitals

now have the oxygen supply piped to the bedside. A flowmeter is attached to the wall fitment and the same precautions apply.
Oxygen may be administered in several ways.
1. By disposable polythene mask (various types).
2. By nasal catheters.
3. Into an oxygen tent.

If oxygen is to be administered continuously, it must be humidified, as dry oxygen is irritating to the respiratory tract. When using a mask, however, adequate humidification is usually obtained when the dry oxygen mixes with the fully saturated expired gases.

Oxygen tents

An oxygen tent is a transparent, airtight compartment into which free oxygen flows over ice to prevent the temperature inside the tent from rising above 18°C (65°F). Oxygen tents are made in various sizes to fit over beds or cots, and have an aperture in front through which the patient receives attention, without interruption of the flow of oxygen. The danger of fire or explosion whilst an oxygen tent is in use must again be stressed.

7
The heart and circulation

The heart is one of the vital organs of the body and, where any part of its structure is diseased or disorganized, its function is impaired and the patient becomes ill.

The heart lies behind the sternum and between the lungs. It is pear shaped and is about the size of its owner's fist. The pointed end rests on the diaphragm towards the left side. The heart is divided lengthwise into two distinct halves by a thin wall of muscle tissue called the septum, and *there is no connection between these two halves.* Each side of the heart is divided into two chambers, the upper chamber is called the atrium and the lower chamber the ventricle, so that there is a right and left atrium and a right and left ventricle. Blood flows *into* the atria and *out from* the ventricles. Between the atria and the ventricles are valves which prevent the backward flow of the blood in the heart. On the right side is the tricuspid valve which has three flaps, while on the left side is the bicuspid or mitral valve with two flaps. The openings from the right ventricle into the pulmonary artery and from the left ventricle into the aorta are guarded by the *semilunar valves,* so called because each valve has three halfmoon-shaped flaps.

Circulation through the heart (Fig. 7.1)

Impure blood carrying carbon dioxide is collected from the lower part of the body by the *inferior vena cava* and from the upper part of the body by the *superior vena cava,* two of the largest veins in the body, and is passed into the right atrium. From the right atrium it passes through the tricuspid valve into the right ventricle, then out of the right ventricle into the pulmonary artery which carries the blood to the lungs, where it gives off carbon dioxide and picks up oxygen. After leaving the lungs the blood is taken into the left atrium by the four pulmonary veins. It then passes through the mitral valve into the left ventricle from where it is pumped into the aorta, to be carried all round the body to nourish the tissues.

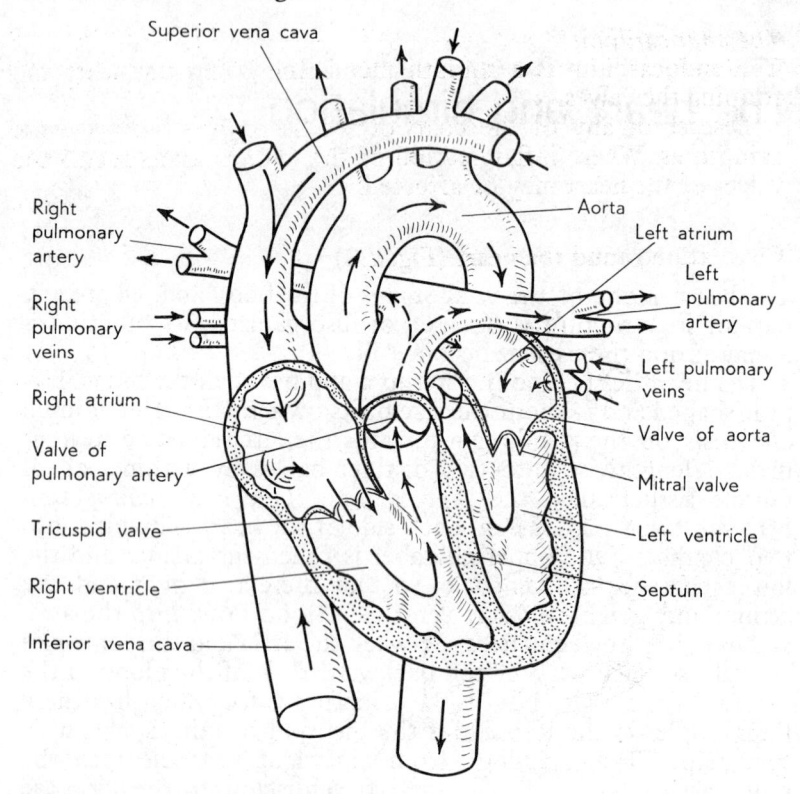

Fig. 7.1 Circulation through the heart.

Formation of the heart

The heart has three coats.

The pericardium
The pericardium, or outer coat, is made up of tough fibrous tissue on its outer surface and serous membrane on the inner surface. The serous membrane secretes a fluid which acts as a lubricant and enables the heart to beat smoothly without friction.

The myocardium
The myocardium is the middle, muscular coat of the heart. This thick, muscular coat is responsible for the rhythmic beat of the heart throughout life.

The endocardium

The endocardium is a smooth membrane lining the heart and forming the valves.

Disease of any of the coats of the heart gives rise to severe symptoms. Where inflammation of the endocardium occurs the valves of the heart may be affected.

Circulation round the heart (Fig. 7.2)

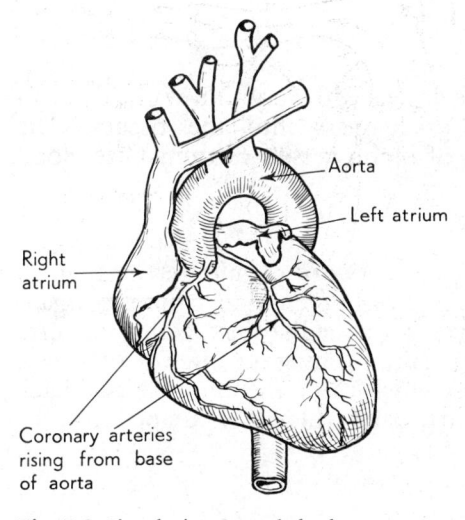

Fig. 7.2 Circulation round the heart.

The tissues of the heart itself are supplied with blood and nourished by the coronary arteries. These vessels rise from the base of the aorta and are contained in grooves on the outer wall of the heart, from where they give off smaller branches. Impure blood from the heart tissues is collected by the coronary veins and poured directly into the right atrium.

Circulation round the body

The blood is carried to every part of the body by a system of blood vessels called *arteries*, *capillaries* and *veins*.

Arteries

Arteries carry oxygenated blood away from the heart to supply the tissues of the body with nourishment and oxygen. (The oxygen is absorbed by the haemoglobin in the red blood cells. See p. 52). The arteries have tough, elastic walls which expand and contract as blood is pumped through them with every beat of the heart, to force the blood round the body in a wave-like motion. Where an artery crosses a bone this movement of blood in the vessel can be felt as the pulse.

N.B. The only artery in the body carrying *venous* blood is the pulmonary artery which takes blood from the right ventricle to the lungs. It will be remembered that the right side of the heart is filled with venous blood.

Capillaries
Capillaries are tiny hair-like vessels with very thin walls, through which nourishment can easily pass into the tissues. The capillaries form a network of blood vessels carrying pure blood to every part of the body.

Veins
In the tissues there is another network of minute veins which collect waste matter, including carbon dioxide, from the organs of the body. These tiny veins gradually join together to form larger and larger veins, eventually forming the *inferior vena cava* and the *superior vena cava*, which carry the impure blood back to the right side of the heart, from where it is pumped into the lungs to be purified (see p. 51).

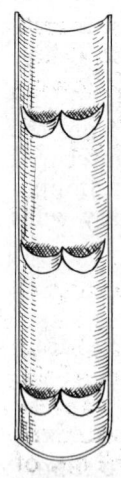

Fig. 7.3 Diagram of formation of veins

The walls of the veins are thinner than those of the arteries and not as strong. The longer veins have valves (Fig. 7.3), shaped like small pockets, along their length to prevent the backward flow of blood in the vessel on its way upwards towards the heart. Where these valves become weakened the venous blood tends to fall backward and collect in the vein causing pain, swelling and discoloration, a condition commonly seen in the lower limbs and known as varicosed veins.

The principal veins of the body follow much the same plan as that of the arteries and usually take the same names: the exceptions are shown in Fig. 7.4.

Haemorrhage

Haemorrhage is the escape of blood from the vessels which carry it round the body.

Primary haemorrhage occurs at the time of injury or operation.

Reactionary haemorrhage occurs within twenty-four hours of injury or operation *after shock has subsided.* As the patient recovers from shock, the blood pressure rises and blood is pumped through the arteries with increasing force until it bursts through a weakened vessel.

Secondary haemorrhage occurs after twenty-four hours and usually within forty-eight hours, but may occur as late as ten to fourteen days after operation. It may be due to sepsis or to a slipped ligature when a blood vessel contracts.

In all cases of suspected haemorrhage the ward sister or staff nurse in charge of the ward must be notified without delay.

Haemorrhage may be due to disease, to injury or following operation. There may be *external haemorrhage* which can be seen outside the body, or *internal haemorrhage* which may be *visible* or *concealed.*

External haemorrhage

There are three types of external haemorrhage according to the blood vessels involved.

1. *Arterial haemorrhage* is bleeding from an artery. The blood is bright red and is forced out in spurts with every beat of the heart. Such bleeding is extremely serious and no time must be lost in dealing with it. In the postoperative care of amputations of limbs, a tourniquet should be attached to the bedrail out of sight of the patient, for use in such an emergency. The bed

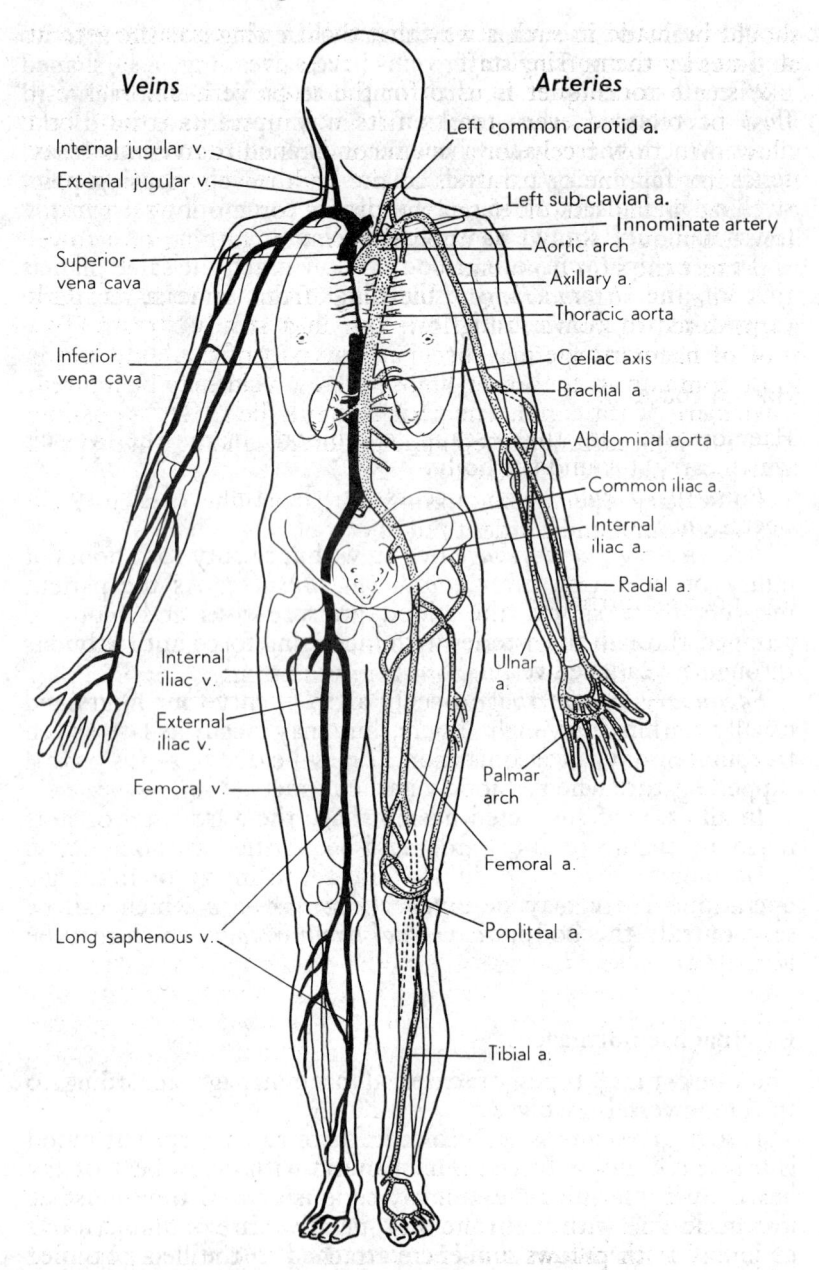

Fig. 7.4 Chief arteries and veins of the body.

should be made in such a way that the dressing is easily seen at all times by the nursing staff.

Where a tourniquet is used for the arrest of haemorrhage it *must* be released every ten to fifteen minutes and the blood allowed to flow freely for a few seconds. Failure to do this may result in gangrene or paralysis of the limb owing to the supply of blood being cut off from the tissues for too long a period. The tourniquet should be applied over the clothing or a towel to protect the skin from injury.

2. *Venous haemorrhage*, bleeding from a vein, is dark purplish-red in colour and flows out in a steady stream. This type of haemorrhage may occur in any part of the body, but is most common in the lower limbs where a vein may be injured, particularly if varicosed. The patient should lie as flat as possible with the injured limb raised and supported, and a firm pad and bandage applied to the bleeding part.

3. *Capillary haemorrhage* oozes out from the capillaries all over the wound and is bright red in colour.

Internal haemorrhage

Internal haemorrhage, whether visible or concealed, may be recognized by the following signs and symptoms.

Extreme pallor of the skin.
Increasingly rapid pulse rate.
Sighing respirations or persistent yawning.
Restlessness and anxiety.
Thirst.
Faintness with gradual loss of consciousness.

Types of visible internal haemorrhage
Epistaxis (bleeding from the nose)   The patient should sit upright and the nostrils should be firmly pinched between thumb and forefinger. The blood will eventually clot. The patient should be warned not to blow the nose and to breathe through the mouth. The nurse must stay with and reassure the patient until the bleeding ceases.

Haemoptysis   Haemoptysis is coughing up of blood from the lungs. The blood is bright red and frothy, because it is mixed with oxygen from the air sacs in the lungs. The patient is usually very frightened and must be reassured whilst being placed in the position found to be most comfortable, well supported with pillows and encouraged to lie as still as possible.

Haematemesis   Haematemesis is bleeding from the stomach.

The vomited blood is dark brown with the appearance of coffee grounds, caused by the action of the gastric juices in the stomach acting on the escaping blood. The patient must be kept very quiet and nothing must be given by mouth.

Haematuria Haematuria is blood in the urine indicating bleeding from the kidney or some part of the urinary passages. The urine may be bright red or clouded in appearance.

Melaena Melaena is blood in the faeces due to haemorrhage in the upper part of the colon. The stool is large, black and shiny, with the appearance of tar.

Haematoma Haematoma is bleeding under the skin, often as a result of a direct below. The blood collects to form a dark swelling under the skin.

Concealed internal haemorrhage
Haemorrhage remains concealed where there is bleeding from the liver, spleen or pancreas. The blood is unable to find an outlet and collects in the abdominal cavity. It can be detected only by the signs and symptoms of haemorrhage shown by the patient (see p. 65).

Concealed haemorrhage may also rise as a result of a complicated fracture, where there is bleeding into the tissues.

Treatment of internal haemorrhage
In all cases of suspected haemorrhage, senior nursing staff must be notified without delay. Speed is essential if the patient's life is to be saved. Screen the bed and raise the foot of the bed on blocks or a bed elevator and remove pillows to allow the patient to lie as flat as possible. The patient must be kept warm but not overheated.

Some common diseases of the heart and blood vessels

General principles of nursing care

Patients suffering from diseases of the heart and blood vessels require careful and skilful nursing.

These patients are nursed in the position in which they are most comfortable, usually in the upright position for those suffering from chronic heart diseases and the recumbent or semi-recumbent for those with acute heart failure.

Extreme care must be taken to prevent bed-sores. Where oedema is present the limbs should be protected with a bed cradle and the feet supported by a pillow or sandbags. The diet should be light and nourishing; a strict intake and output chart recorded and all urine measured. The rate, rhythm and volume of the pulse are important guides in the observation and nursing of all diseases of the heart and circulatory system and are taken and recorded four-hourly or more frequently where ordered. Oxygen should be kept within easy reach of the bed in case of emergency. Restlessness and anxiety are common symptoms, and constant comfort, reassurance and freedom from anxiety are important to the recovery of the patient. It is the nurse who has the opportunity of giving this reassurance, being the person who works close to such ill people, and the one to whom they will turn in their distress. At no time should the impression be given that there is too little time to spend with the patient.

Pericarditis

Pericarditis is inflammation of the pericardium, the outer covering of the heart. The danger of this disease is that the inflammation may spread to the muscular wall of the heart (the myocardium). The patient complains of pain in the chest and may become restless and distressed. The pulse is rapid, irregular, with an irregular swinging temperature and dyspnoea. Hot local applications such as kaolin poultice may be ordered for the relief of pain.

Myocarditis

Myocarditis is inflammation of the muscular wall of the heart and may be chronic or acute. This may be the result of the spread of inflammation from one of the other coats of the heart, either the pericardium, as described above, or of the endocardium. The heart muscle becomes flabby and loses some of its power. This affects the pulse rate which becomes rapid and irregular.

Endocarditis

Endocarditis is inflammation of the membrane lining the heart. In this instance the valves of the heart may be involved because they are continuous with the endocardium. Endocarditis may be the result of such infectious diseases as measles, scarlet fever or rheumatic fever. Often the heart disease does not become evident until many years after the initial illness.

Mitral stenosis

Mitral stenosis is a narrowing of the opening of the mitral valve between the left atrium and the left ventricle and may be the result of endocarditis.

Chronic congestive heart disease

This has a wide variety of causes. The heart muscle weakens and the heart becomes enlarged. The pumping action is affected and the circulation is impaired. The patient often suffers some respiratory distress (dyspnoea) and develops a cough with expectoration of sputum. The renal system may be affected also and the output of urine is lessened. Other symptoms include cyanosis, oedema, faintness, giddiness, fluttering and throbbing sensations in the chest and enlargement of the liver.

Coronary thrombosis

Coronary thrombosis occurs as a result of some part of the coronary artery being blocked by a clot of blood and the supply of blood to the heart is reduced or cut off. Even while resting in bed the patient may have an attack of pain spreading over the chest and shoulder and down the arm, accompanied by all the signs and symptoms of shock (see p. 233). During an attack the patient must not be left alone and must be reassured. Patients are mobilized as soon as possible, depending on the severity of the attack.

Angina pectoris

Angina pectoris is also due to some defect in the coronary artery resulting in an insufficient supply of blood to the walls of the heart, particularly the myocardium. An attack may occur when the patient is working, taking unaccustomed exercise or on a display of violent emotion such as anger. Acute pain is felt across the pectoral muscle covering the left front side of the chest and spreading down the arm.

Arteriosclerosis

Arteriosclerosis is the term used to describe the hardening of the arteries. The walls of the arteries lose their elasticity and become thickened, with the result that the blood has less space in the vessels in which to circulate. This gives rise to high blood pressure (hypertension) a condition often associated with advancing age. The pulse is full and bounding and the face usually appears flushed.

Thrombosis

Thrombosis is clotting of blood in a blood vessel, commonly where there is inflammation of the inner coat of an artery or vein.

Embolism

Embolism is a clot or part of a clot of blood which becomes detached and travels in the bloodstream. An embolus may also consist of air, fat or small fragments of free floating tissue, all of which may lodge in an artery.

Phlebitis

Phlebitis is inflammation of a vein. It may be the result of injury, infectious disease or following childbirth. The chief danger in a deep vein is the formation of a blood clot over the inflamed area which may become dislodged and travel round the body to block a vital centre such as the brain, heart or lung, and prove fatal. Patients having a suspected phlebitis must be nursed with the utmost care to lessen the risk of an embolus breaking away into the general circulation.

Measurement of blood pressure

Blood pressure means the tension of blood in the arteries. The pressure depends on the strength of the heart beat, the elasticity of the coats of the arteries, the amount of fluid circulating in the body and the ability of the small arteries (arterioles) to close down when fluids are lost from the body. Blood pressure is measured with a sphygmomanometer in millimetres of mercury (often written as mmHg). This instrument consists of a rubber bag in a cotton cover with a hand pump attached. As air is pumped into the bag the mercury in the manometer rises to indicate the pressure.

When taking the blood pressure the patient should be sitting or lying down. The manometer should be placed so that the patient cannot see the mercury rising.

The rubber bag is wrapped smoothly round the arm about

2.5 cm (1 in) above the elbow and the ends tucked in firmly. Keeping the fingers on the pulse at the wrist, air is pumped into the bag. When the pulse can no longer be felt, the valve on the hand pump is slowly opened and the fall of mercury watched until the pulse at the wrist can again be felt. The figure registered on the manometer at this point must be noted. This is the *systolic blood pressure*.

A more exact estimation of the blood pressure can be obtained by the use of a stethoscope applied over the brachial artery at the bend of the elbow. A muffled sound will be heard. The bag is inflated until the sound disappears. The valve on the pump is opened and the mercury allowed to fall slowly. When tapping sounds can be heard the level of the mercury should be noted. This is the systolic pressure.

The mercury is allowed to fall still further and the sounds become louder. When these loud sounds change to the muffled sound originally heard, the level of the mercury in the manometer must be noted again. This is the *diastolic* blood pressure.

The systolic blood pressure is the highest point registered by the mercury when the heart contracts and the arteries are filled with blood. The diastolic pressure is the lowest point registered on the manometer during the resting stage of the heart.

The normal blood pressure of an adult is approximately 120/75 millimetres of mercury. The first figure is the systolic pressure and the second figure the diastolic pressure. Blood pressure increases with age and is higher for men than for women.

8
The blood

Normal blood consists of two parts: a clear, yellowish fluid known as plasma, and a more solid part made up of red and white cells and platelets. The body contains about 5 litres (or 9 pints) of blood.

Plasma
Plasma is made up of about 92 per cent water and carries mineral salts, proteins and sugars to nourish the tissues. Excess nourishment not needed immediately by the tissues is passed into the lymphatic vessels (see p. 112).

Red blood cells
Red blood cells are tiny, biconcave discs which are manufactured in bone marrow. They contain a coloured pigment called *haemoglobin* which, with its iron, carries oxygen to the tissues. In health the red blood cells number about 5 million per cubic millimetre.

White blood cells
White blood cells, or leucocytes, are known as the defenders of the body because they attack and attempt to destroy germs which may gain entry. These cells have the power of movement and can squeeze themselves through capillary walls into the tissues. They are larger than the red cells and not so numerous, in health varying between 7000 and 10 000 per cubic millimetre.

Platelets
Platelets are tiny bodies, smaller than the red cells. They assist in the clotting of blood by coagulation, thus arresting haemorrhage.

For diagnostic purposes, a specimen of the patient's blood may be sent to the pathological laboratory for examination. An important test is the blood count which gives the number of red and white cells in the blood and the amount of haemoglobin present.

Blood grouping and transfusion

Normal blood contains certain factors which are responsible for different blood groups. In the classification of human blood, people are divided into four groups according to the factors in the blood stream. Some have A blood grouping, some have B and some have both factors AB. These groups cannot be mixed because the blood serum from one group will cause the red cells of another group to stick together and form clots in the body which would have extremely serious consequences and may result in the death of a patient. The fourth group (O) does not react to other groups and can be given to almost all other people without ill effect. People with group O blood are referred to as universal donors.

There is another factor called the Rhesus factor. Where present, the blood is said to be Rhesus positive (Rh +) and if absent Rhesus negative (Rh-). This factor is especially important in obstetrics. The blood from donors most frequently used is Group O Rh +.

In every case of transfusion the donor's blood is cross-matched against that of the recipient. Matched units of blood must be labelled clearly with the full name and age of the patient, ABO and Rhesus grouping, the name of the ward and the patient's case number. The serial number of the unit also appears on the label. All this information must be carefully checked at the bedside, according to hospital policy. The nurse has a great responsibility when handling blood: mistakes can lead to tragedy. Special care must be taken when more than one blood transfusion is in progress at the same time. Before commencing a subsequent unit the same stringent checking procedure must be adopted.

The equipment required for a transfusion is the same as for an intravenous infusion (p. 124). A giving set incorporating a filter must be used. The rate of flow will be decided by the doctor. Strict watch must be kept on the drip chamber. If it becomes full or the rate of flow changes, the ward sister must be informed without delay. The tubing must not be allowed to kink or the flow will cease and care must be taken that when making the bed, the tubing is not pulled or pinched. The nurse should report when a container is almost empty.

During a blood transfusion the patient must be closely

observed for an signs of rigor, twitching, nausea, vomiting or irregular pulse. These are the signs of reaction to the blood and must be reported at once.

Most patients are aware that intravenous fluids, including blood, are in common use. Nevertheless, some patients (and their visitors) become alarmed when they see the intravenous apparatus, especially if blood is being given. The nurse should make every effort to give the reassurance that the procedure is to hasten recovery. Where possible, the drip stand should be placed out of the line of vision of the patient.

Whole blood is given to replace extensive loss of blood due to haemorrhage which results in a reduction of red cells, haemoglobin and oxygen in the body (see p. 71).

Packed cells. This is blood from which some of the plasma has been removed. This is used where extra haemoglobin is needed without increasing the amount of blood in the body and is often used in the treatment of severe anaemia.

Plasma may be separated from whole blood and dried. When required for use, distilled water is added. Plasma increases the blood volume and contributes protein and is used in the treatment of shock or where there is severe loss of body fluids other than blood. Plasma protein substitute is also available ready for use.

Some common diseases of the blood

Anaemia

By this term is meant a deficiency in the number or quality of red blood cells, which may be due to an insufficient supply of the substances needed by the blood, such as iron or haemoglobin. Symptoms vary, but the patient usually complains of a general feeling of illness with loss of appetite, headache, dyspnoea or tachycardia (abnormally rapid heart beat). Pallor of the mucous membrane of the lower eyelids or lips is a common sign of anaemia.

Erratum
Forrest and Watson: **Practical Nursing and Anatomy for Pupil Nurses 4th Edition**
p. 72, line 20
For 'Group O Rh+'
read 'Group O Rhesus negative (Rh-)'.

symptoms of anaemia are present. The onset is gradual and there may be muscular weakness which will develop into exhaustion unless treated. Sore mouth and gums, vomiting and nausea, oedema of the ankles or eyelids and pyrexia at intervals are further signs and symptoms which may arise according to the severity of the disease. A good nourishing diet is essential with plenty of foods containing iron (see p. 90). Intramuscular injections of vitamin B_{12} may be ordered to be given once or twice weekly.

Leukaemia

The outstanding feature of this disease is the great increase in the number of white blood cells or leucocytes. The cause is unknown but is believed to be due to some defect in those organs concerned with the manufacture of the white cells, i.e. the spleen or lymphatic glands. The disease may start suddenly or may be a complication of severe illness. Common signs and symptoms are bleeding from the gums, fatigue and debility.

Inflammation

Inflammation may be local or general and occurs as a result of injury or of the entry into the body of bacteria.

Inflammation is not in itself a disease, but is a sign that the tissues are resisting attack by harmful bacteria capable of producing toxins or poisons in the bloodstream.

In order to fight off this bacterial invasion, the blood vessels dilate to allow more blood to flow to the affected part, bringing with it a greater stream of white cells, which are the defence system of the body. They surround the germs and attempt to kill them by breaking down and absorbing them.

Where the infection is slight, the white cells return to the bloodstream after killing the bacteria and the inflammation dies down. If the germs are the stronger, many of the white cells are destroyed and become semi-fluid. With the dead and living bacteria and their toxins, together with fragments of dead tissue, a semi-solid substance is formed, called pus, which eventually finds its way to the surface of the affected organ.

In an attempt to prevent the infection from spreading, the blood has the ability of creating a barrier around the point of entry by the bacteria, so that the infection is controlled within a small area. The tissues in this area become engorged with blood, giving rise to the redness and heat indicating local

inflammation. It is in this way that abscesses are formed.
Signs and symptoms of local inflammation are redness, heat, swelling, throbbing pain and loss of function.
Treatment includes rest of the affected part and hot or cold applications.

General inflammation

This occurs as a result of the toxins or poisons created by the bacteria entering the bloodstream, causing *toxaemia*. If the bacteria themselves enter the bloodstream they give rise to an extremely serious condition known as *septicaemia*, which, unless treated promptly, may prove fatal.

Signs and symptoms of general inflammation are rising temperature, hot, dry skin, headache, coated tongue, thirst and malaise. The nursing care is as for any severe illness and should include complete bed rest, warmth without overheating, plenty of fluids, light, nourishing diet and prevention of constipation.

Hot applications

Poultices

These provide a method of applying heat to an affected area with the advantage of retaining the heat for long periods. The patient therefore need not be disturbed too often.

Requirements for a kaolin poultice
    Tin of kaolin, saucepan of boiling water.
    Lint or old linen, poultice board and palette knife.
    Jug of boiling water in which to stand the palette knife.
    Two warmed plates, cotton wool to cover poultice, bandage and safety pins.
    Olive oil standing in a bowl of warm water; wool swabs; receiver.
    Method Place the tin of kaolin in the saucepan of boiling water and allow it to heat for about twenty minutes, stirring occasionally to mix the oils and to distribute the heat evenly. Cut away the corners of the lint or linen and place on the poultice board. Spread the kaolin with the palette knife about 0.25 cm thick, cover with gauze and turn in the edges to make a neat square. Carry the poultice to the bedside between two warmed plates on a tray, together with the bowl containing the wool, bandage, and olive oil if required. Test the heat of the

poultice with the wrist before applying gently to the skin. Care must be taken when applying these poultices, as they hold the heat to an extensive degree and, if not tested, may result in serious burns. Cover with cotton wool and bandage. If on removing a poultice the skin appears red and sensitive, it may be swabbed with olive oil. Individually packed kaolin poultices are now available. The maufacturer's instructions should be followed.

Cold applications

Inflammation due to injury, such as a sprain, may be treated with cold applications. They help to decrease the circulation of blood to the part, relieving pain, congestion and swelling. They also assist in removing excess heat from the injured part by evaporation through the skin.

Cold compress

Requirements
   Double fold of lint, iced water.
   Forceps; wringer, two bowls.
   Method   The lint is wrung out in the iced water, applied to the affected part and bandaged firmly. The compress should be applied with forceps so that the heat of the hand does not come into contact with it. The application should be changed frequently so that it is kept cold and moist. Reusable cold packs are also now commercially available.

Evaporating compress

This is applied in exactly the same way as the cold compress, using an evaporating agent such as methylated spirit, eau-de-Cologne or a lotion of lead and opium.
   Method   The lint is wrung out in iced water containing the evaporating lotion and is lightly bandaged to the affected part. When applied to a limb, a cradle should be used to allow a free current of air to circulate in order to promote the rapid removal of heat from the injured part.

9
The urinary system

The kidneys

The kidneys form part of the excretory or urinary system. (Fig. 9.1). They are two dark red, bean-shaped organs, situated one on each side of the backbone in the lumbar region, and are surrounded by a mass of fatty tissue which forms a means of protection. The kidneys are outside the peritoneum, which covers most of the other abdominal organs.

The tissue of the kidneys is well supplied with tiny blood vessels which pass waste matter from the body into a system of small tubes. This waste matter is then passed into the pelvis of

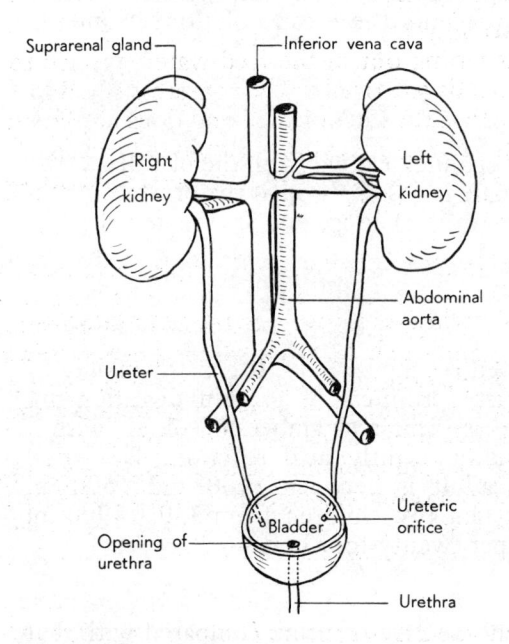

Fig. 9.1 The urinary system.

the kidney from where it is poured into the ureters as urine.

The kidneys also assist in regulating the balance of fluids in the body. If there is too much fluid in the tissues, more urine will normally be excreted: if too little is present in the body, the kidneys are not so active and waste matter is not efficiently excreted. Where the kidneys become diseased and unable to function properly waste matter remains in the bloodstream causing severe illness, such as uraemia.

The ureters

The ureters are two fine tubes, about 25-30 cm (10-12 in) long, one from each kidney, connecting it with the bladder.

The bladder

The bladder is a hollow muscular organ, lined with mucous membrane, which acts as a reservoir for urine until it is excreted. The bladder lies within the pelvic cavity until full, then it rises into the abdominal cavity. The external opening is guarded by a tight ring of muscle, called a sphincter, which is under voluntary control and prevents the escape of urine from the bladder.

The urethra

The urethra is a narrow channel leading from the bladder to the external orifice. In the male it passes through the prostate gland, and is about 15-20 cm (6-8 in) long, and in the female it is about 4 cm long.

Urine

Urine is the fluid excreted by the kidneys. It consists mainly of water in which the waste products of protein digestion are dissolved. Normal urine is clear and amber in colour, with a characteristic odour and a slightly acid reaction. The usual amount passed by an adult is between 1100 and 1500 ml (40 to 50 fluid ounces) and by children from 350 to 900 ml (12 to 30 fluid ounces) per twenty-four hours.

Specific gravity
The specific gravity is the density of urine compared with that of water, which is taken as 1000. The normal specific gravity of

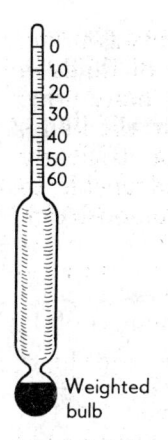

Fig. 9.2 Urinometer.

urine is from 1015 to 1025 and is measured with a urinometer (Fig. 9.2) during routine ward examination.

Deposits
Abnormal urine may appear cloudy or contain deposits which may be due to pus, blood, mucus, phosphates or urates. If the urine is allowed to stand, these abnormalities will appear as sediment at the bottom of the specimen glass. The nurse must inspect all urine before disposal and report any abnormalities which may be evident. It must be measured and recorded when required.

Special terms and their meanings

Micturition is the passing of urine from the bladder.

Frequency of micturition is the frequent passing of small amounts of urine.

Incontinence of urine is the inability to retain urine owing to some weakness of the sphincter guarding the outlet from the bladder.

Retention of urine is due to the inability to pass urine so that the bladder becomes overfull, causing abdominal distension. Catheterization may be ordered to relieve this condition.

Retention with incontinence occurs when the bladder becomes so full and distended that the urine is forced out by pressure. This condition may also be relieved by catheterization.

Suppression of urine is due to failure of the kidneys to

function efficiently in the production of urine. Waste matter is retained and circulated in the bloodstream instead of being excreted and the patient becomes extremely ill.

Enuresis. This is the involuntary passing of urine during sleep, as in childhood.

Dysuria is painful micturition.

Urine testing

Examination of urine is an important part of the nurse's duties, and must be accurate. The urine of all new patients is fully tested on admission and routine tests are taken before all operations, for diagnostic purposes or to estimate any change in the condition of the patient. The results of the tests are reported and recorded each time they are carried out.

To collect a specimen of urine: the patient is given a clean bedpan or urinal before breakfast. The urine is poured into a clean specimen glass labelled with the patient's name and the date.

A 24-hour specimen of urine consists of all urine passed during a period of twenty-four hours. On the morning of the first day the patient is given a bedpan or urinal at a stated hour and the urine is thrown away. All urine passed after this hour is collected and placed in a covered vessel clearly labelled with the patient's name and the date. The last specimen is taken at the same hour on the following morning and added to the rest. This completes a 24-hour specimen of urine. The test may be made from a sample; the urine is stirred with a glass rod in order to distribute the deposits evenly and a specimen poured off for testing. Where the whole amount is to be examined, the vessel containing the urine is sent to the pathological laboratory for investigation.

A catheter specimen is sterile. The urine is drawn off from the bladder under aseptic conditions and sent to the pathological laboratory for examination.

Routine ward examination of urine

The specific gravity is taken first.

The Ames Company reagent strips and tablets have now made urine testing very simple, but the manufacturer's instructions concerning both the chemical testing and also the storage of the reagents and tablets must be strictly followed for accurate results.

Test for protein Albustix

Test for protein Albustix
Dip the test end of an Albustix into the urine and remove immediately. Compare the colour of the test-end with the colour chart provided with the Albustix. If the moistened end turns green at once, albumin is present. Where the colour remains yellow, albumin is absent.

Albumin in urine (albuminuria) usually occurs in renal disease and sometimes in pregnancy.

Tests for sugar

Clinistix
This is a test for glucose only. The reagent strip is dipped in the specimen of urine and read after sixty seconds. If glucose is present, this turns blue. Urine reacting positively to this test should be further tested by the following method.

Clinitest
This is a more accurate test and is the one used for diabetic patients.

Five drops of urine and then ten drops of water are dropped into a clean testtube specially provided for these tests. One clinitest tablet is added and, fifteen seconds after boiling has ceased, the tube is shaken and the colour of the fluid is compared with the colour chart. The colours range from blue to green and orange and represent a range of 0% to 2% sugar. It must be noted, however, that, if at any stage of the test an orange colour appears, the result is recorded as 2% irrespective of the final colour.

Tests for ketones

Acetest
Place 1 Acetest tablet on a piece of clean white paper. Put 1 drop of urine on the tablet and wait *exactly* thirty seconds. Compare the result with the colour chart provided. If the tablet remains white or cream, the test is negative. Ketones are present if the tablet turns mauve.

Tests for sugar (glucose), diacetic acid or acetone and ketones are conducted where there is suspected or diagnosed diabetes mellitus or disease of the pancreas.

Test for blood

Urine with blood in it is called *haematuria*, but only if present in a large quantity can it be seen with the naked eye.

Hemastix

Stir the urine with a glass rod. Dip the test end of a Hemastix strip into the urine and remove it immediately. Wait thirty seconds and then compare the colour of the test end of the strip with the colour chart. If blood is present, the test end will turn blue within thirty seconds. Where no blood is present the test strip remains off white at thirty seconds. Any colour appearing after this time should be ignored. Blood in urine may be detected in diseases of the genitourinary tract.

Tests for bile

Ictotest

Place 5 drops of urine on the square test mat provided and put 1 Ictotest tablet in the centre of the moist area. Place 2 drops of water on the tablet and wait for thirty seconds. If bile is present, the test mat around the tablet will turn a bluish-purple within thirty seconds. If no colour appears on the mat at thirty seconds or it turns faintly red or orange, the result is negative.

The presence of bile in urine indicates disease of the liver, bile ducts or gall bladder. Bile salts are usually present in cases of obstructive jaundice.

Intake and output charting

In certain illnesses it is important to keep a strict record of the quantity of fluid taken and excreted by the patient. All fluids taken, whether by mouth, rectum, or intravenously, are recorded in one column of the intake and output chart, and all fluids excreted such as urine, vomitus, watery stools or fluid taken off by aspiration, are recorded in another column (Fig. 9.3). At the end of the day the two columns are added separately and the balance of fluid is obtained by deducting one total from the other. The total intake should exceed the output by about 900 ml (30 oz), unless this is contra-indicated by the condition of the patient, as in oedema where there is too much fluid in the tissues. If the output is greater than the intake, there may be a danger of the patient becoming dehydrated, i.e. lack of body fluids. A certain amount of fluid is lost during respiration

DATE	TIME	INTAKE: ORAL	INTAKE: RECTAL	INTAKE: INTRAVENOUS Remarks	INTAKE: INTRAVENOUS Amount Given	OUTPUT: Gastric Aspiration	OUTPUT: URINE	OUTPUT: Other routes	OUTPUT: REMARKS
	8 a.m.								
	9 a.m.								
	10 a.m.								
	11 a.m.								
	12 noon								
	1 p.m.								
	2 p.m.								
	3 p.m.								
	4 p.m.								
	5 p.m.								
	6 p.m.								
	7 p.m.								
	8 p.m.								
	9 p.m.								
	10 p.m.								
	11 p.m.								
	12 m'nt								
	1 a.m.								
	2 a.m.								
	3 a.m.								
	4 a.m.								
	5 a.m.								
	6 a.m.								
	7 a.m.								
	8 a.m.								
TOTALS									INSENSIBLE LOSS 1000 ml.
		TOTAL INTAKE				TOTAL OUTPUT			

Fig. 9.3 Fluid intake and output chart.

and by the action of the sweat glands in the skin. This cannot be measured and is known as insensible loss. The amount lost is estimated at 1000 ml each twenty-four hours.

Catheterization

Catheterization means the withdrawal of urine from the bladder by artificial means, through the urethra. Various types of disposable catheters are available for the purpose. When the catheter is to be left in the bladder, a self-retaining type is used. These are balloon ended and the balloon is inflated once the catheter is in situ, thus preventing displacement.

Reasons for catheterization

To relieve retention of urine.
Before operation.

84 Practical nursing

To obtain specimens of urine for diagnostic purposes.

When other methods of collection are impossible, as during incontinence.

To administer treatment to the bladder.

To ascertain the amount of residual urine, i.e. the urine left in the bladder after normal micturition.

Catheterization must be performed using a strict aseptic technique as there is a serious risk of introducing infection into the bladder.

Catheter trolley for female patient
 Top shelf
  Sterile pack containing:
   dressing towels or aperture towel;
   dressing forceps;
   gallipot;
   wool balls.

 Bottom shelf
  Cleansing lotion.
  Appropriate catheter.
  Sterile receiver for urine.
  Universal container.
  Laboratory form.
  Sterile gloves.
  Masks.
  Sterile spigot.

  If a self-retaining catheter is used:
   urine drainage bag with holder;
   syringe;
   hypodermic needle;
   ampoule of sterile water;
   adhesive strapping.

  In addition:
   anglepoise lamp.

Preparation of a female patient

Place the patient in the dorsal position if possible. The genitals should be thoroughly washed with soap and water beforehand. Prepare the sterile trolley, as above, screen the bed and close nearby windows. Explain to the patient, in simple language, what is to be done, and that the procedure may be a little uncomfortable but not painful. Assist relaxation by keeping the patient warm and by carrying out the preparation and procedure as quickly, gently and efficiently as possible.

Prepare the bed by turning down the top bed-clothes. Cover the patient's shoulders with a small blanket. Have the patient comfortably in the dorsal position with one or two pillows under the head. Adjust the anglepoise lamp so that it shines directly on the vulva. Wash the hands thoroughly and dry on a sterile towel. Put on sterile gloves. Place a sterile towel over each of the patient's legs, one over the abdomen and one on the bed.

Using an antiseptic, swab the genitals in a downward direction, using each swab once only and discarding it. Leave a swab in the vaginal orifice to prevent contamination. Note any anatomical defect which may make the passage of the catheter difficult.

Place the sterile receiver on the bed between the patient's legs. Pick up the catheter taking care to avoid touching the tip and pass it into the urethra for about 5 cm (2 in) or until urine flows. If the specimen is required for the pathological laboratory, discard the first few millilitres, then pass the end of the catheter into a sterile specimen jar with forceps. While the bladder is being emptied the nurse's hand should rest firmly over the lower abdomen to control the collapsing bladder. This helps to lessen any feeling of shock the patient may suffer. If the bladder is grossly distended, the urine should be released slowly to prevent shock.

Record and report the amount of urine obtained and note if there was difficulty in passing the catheter.

Male catheterization

Male nursing or medical staff are usually responsible for carrying out this procedure. Strict aseptic precautions must be taken to prevent infection. The procedure should be explained to the patient and reassurance given.

Bladder washout

The bladder may be washed out to prevent the formation of blood clots after operation on the bladder, or as treatment for the mucous membrane lining the bladder, as in cases of chronic cystitis. A bladder syringe with a rubber bulb is usually found to be most satisfactory, as the pressure of the irrigating fluid is easily controlled and good suction is obtained, both important points in efficient treatment and the comfort of the patient. A bladder washout is a sterile procedure.

Some common diseases of the urinary system

Nephritis
Nephritis is inflammation of the kidney and may be acute or chronic.

Acute nephritis
Acute nephritis is often a complication of other diseases such as scarlet fever, tonsillitis or severe burns, particularly of the abdomen.

The onset is sudden with rigor, pyrexia, vomiting and oedema of the face, especially of the eyelids. The output of urine is diminished and albumin or blood may be present in the urine.

Nursing treatment The patient is initially on complete bed rest and all unnecessary movement avoided. Extra warmth should be provided and a daily blanket bath given to encourage efficient excretion of waste matter by the sweat glands, thus helping to relieve some of the strain on the affected kidneys. Pressure areas should be treated and the position of the patient changed at frequent intervals.

Diet is important in the treatment of acute nephritis. Because the whole kidney is affected and its function seriously impaired, very little urine is passed. For this reason proteins are usually restricted until recovery is established. If oedema is marked, fluids and salts in the diet may also be restricted. The urine should be tested daily for albumin and the results recorded. An accurate fluid chart must be kept and checked daily.

Chronic nephritis
Chronic nephritis is a disease which may last for years. The signs and symptoms vary according to the progress of the disease. Patients suffering from chronic nephritis show signs of oedema at some time during the course of the disease, and in the last

stages the signs and symptoms are the same as those of uraemia, e.g. vomiting, suppression of urine and coma.

The patient should be kept very warm and have a well-balance diet with plenty of proteins and fluids, but where oedema is evident, fluids and salt in the diet may be restricted. Patients suffering from renal failure, either acute or chronic, may have waste substances removed from the body by means of peritoneal or haemodialysis.

Pyelitis

Pyelitis is inflammation of the pelvis of the kidney and may be due to infection by staphylococci, streptococci or to the *Escherichia coli*. It is a common disease which may occur in infancy and during pregnancy. The onset of pyelitis is sudden, with pyrexia, rigor and frequency of micturition, accompanied by pain.

Nursing treatment
The patient is nursed as for any severe illness, on bed rest, with a light, nourishing diet, including plenty of fluids. All pressure areas should be treated at regular intervals, care being taken that the patient does not become chilled. Where rigors occur they must be treated as described on page 24. The urine is tested daily for albumin and pus, and an intake and output chart kept.

Pyelitis is not to be confused with nephritis. Pyelitis is an inflammation of the pelvis of the kidney, while nephritis is inflammation of the substance of the kidney.

Cystitis

Cystitis is inflammation of the mucous membrane lining the bladder, occurring more often in female than in males. It is a painful condition causing frequency of micturition with pain. The urine may contain albumin, or pus, and in acute cases pyrexia and rigor may occur. This condition may be caused by repeated or careless catheterizations. The need for the utmost care in catheterization cannot be stressed too strongly.

Nursing care
Nursing care includes warmth, a light, nourishing diet and reassurance. A patient suffering from cystitis should never be kept waiting for a bedpan, even though the amount of urine passed is consistently small. Neither should impatience be shown with the constant demands of such a patient. Anxiety will aggravate the condition and retard recovery, and must be avoided as much as possible.

10
Food, diets and digestion

Food
Food is required to maintain the normal functions of the body and to build and repair body tissues which are constantly being broken down, in health as well as in disease. Before food can enter the tissues it must be changed into simple substances which can pass easily into the bloodstream. The changes in food brought about by the digestive process are described on page 101.

Metabolism
The breaking down and rebuilding of body tissues, the giving off of waste matter and the production and loss of heat and energy is known as *metabolism*. The same process taking place while the body is at rest is known as *basal metabolism*. Food is divided into the following six essential factors, all of which should be included in the well-balanced diet. In certain diseases, it may become necessary to omit one or more of the food factors.

1. *Proteins* are the body-building foods necessary for the repair and growth of the tissues. They are constituents of meat, fish, eggs, milk and cheese, peas, beans and nuts. During digestion, proteins are broken down into substances called amino acids which are taken into the bloodstream and used by the body to form new proteins.

2. *Carbohydrates*, such as starches and sugars, are stores of heat and energy. Starch is contained in flour, bread, potatoes and cereals. Sugars are to be found in jam, sweets, honey, sugar and beetroot. During digestion, carbohydrates including starches are changed into glucose and stored in the liver until needed. Glucose is one of the simplest forms of sugar and is easily absorbed into the bloodstream.

3. *Fats* also provide heat and energy, but less fat is needed

for this purpose than carbohydrate. Examples of fatty foods are butter, cream, margarine, olive oil, fat meat and fat fish such as herring and salmon. During the digestive process fats are reduced to oily substances known as fatty acids and glycerol.

4. *Mineral salts* are necessary for the healthy formation of teeth and bones, and the efficient action of nerves, glands and organs of the body. A sufficient amount of each is provided in the normal diet.

(*a*) *Calcium and phosphorus* are required for the formation of teeth and bones, the clotting of blood and the smooth working of the muscles, including the heart muscle. These salts are especially important for the normal growth and development of babies and children. The chief sources of *calcium* are milk, cheese, fish and green vegetables; and of *phosphorus*, meat meat, fish, eggs and oatmeal.

(*b*) *Iron* is needed by the red blood cells and is found in red meat, liver, eggs, green vegetables, dried fruit and cocoa.

(*c*) *Sodium chloride* is common salt and is widely distributed among all classes of food, and is contained in body fluids.

(*d*) *Iodine* found in sea foods, is needed by the thyroid gland.

(*e*) *Sulphur* is needed for growth of body cells.

5. *Water* is essential to life and should be taken freely to replace loss of body fluids, as sweat, urine, in faeces and in breath.

6. *Vitamins* are complicated chemical substances essential for the maintenance of health. They are present in small amounts in foodstuffs, and an ordinary mixed diet will contain enough vitamins for the needs of the body. Where the diet has to be restricted, extra vitamins are given.

Vitamin A builds resistance to infection and is necessary for growth and development. It is found in milk, butter, cheese and egg yolk and cod liver and halibut liver oils and in green vegetables. Lack of vitamin A may result in respiratory infections because of the lowered resistance of mucous membrane to infection. Eye diseases also arise as a result of lack of this vitamin.

Vitamin B is made up of several factors known as the vitamin B complex, and is concerned with the healthy development of skin, nerves and blood cells. It is found in milk, cheese, eggs, fish, meat, liver and kidneys, cereals, peas and beans and in yeast. Deficiency of vitamin B causes beriberi and is common in eastern countries, where the main article of diet is polished rice from which the vitamin-carrying husk has been removed in the polishing process. Pellagra is another disease due to a lack of vitamin B and gives rise to gastrointestinal and mental disturbances as well as dermatitis of the skin.

Vitamin C (ascorbic acid) is necessary for the growth and repair of tissues and capillary walls. The chief sources of this vitamin are oranges, lemons, blackcurrants, rose hips, green vegetables, tomatoes and potatoes. Boiling destroys vitamin C. Insufficient vitamin C gives rise to scurvy, a disease marked by anaemia, swollen spongy gums, haemorrhages into the skin (purpura), epistaxis and a general feeling of illness. Small babies being artifically fed need vitamin C in the form of multivitamin drops or orange juice after 1 month of age. The vitamin content of dried milk should be taken into consideration. Breast-fed babies rarely contract scurvy because there is normally sufficient vitamin C in human milk to safeguard the child against this disease.

Vitamin D is found in foods with vitamin A. It controls the use of calcium in the formation of bones and teeth. The main sources of vitamin D are cod liver oil, halibut liver oil, dairy produce and animal fats. Vitamin D is also produced by the action of the sun's rays on the fatty substance in the skin, and can be produced artificially by irradiation with ultraviolet lamps, a method adopted in the manufacture of margarine and other proprietary foodstuffs. *Rickets* (deformity of bones) is caused by lack of vitamin D in food or of sunlight. In the prevention of rickets, cod liver and halibut liver oils may be added to the diet of children.

Vitamin E is sometimes called the anti-sterility vitamin because it is believed to prevent abortion. It is contained in wheat germ.

Vitamin K is needed for the formation of prothrombin, an essential factor in clotting of blood. It is found in spinach, cabbage, cauliflower and oats. Deficiency of vitamin K may result in diseases affecting the digestive system, followed by haemorrhages owing to insufficient prothrombin in the blood.

Roughage consists of the fibrous, undigested parts of fruits and vegetables which are passed into the large intestine in bulk, and is necessary for bodily health and prevention of constipation. This waste matter is passed along the intestines by peristaltic action to be excreted.

Milk

Milk is used extensively in feeding patients because it is easily digested and contains all the food factors needed by the body, i.e. proteins, carbohydrates, fats, mineral salts, vitamins and water. In its raw state it is usually teeming with bacteria, most of which are destroyed by processing as described below. Milk is easily contaminated and can carry disease unless the utmost cleanliness is maintained by all who handle milk and milk containers. It is illegal in Britain to sell milk from diseased cows, or to add water or preservatives to the milk. Dairy farms and farmers must be registered with the Department of Agriculture and cowsheds and milking equipment are inspected periodically by authorized Health Inspectors. The Department of Health can prohibit the sale of milk from farms and other premises where people suffering from infectious disease live or work.

In a well run dairy farm the cowsheds are kept scrupulously clean and have a good supply of running water. The udders and hind quarters of the cows are washed thoroughly before milking, the dirty water draining away into properly constructed channels. The milkers wear clean white coats and caps and all equipment is sterilized before and after use. Facilities are provided where the milkers can wash the hands before commencing milking.

In some instances, a portion of the milk is bottled on the farm, usually by machinery, but the bulk of the milk is collected into dustproof, watertight and sterilized churns or glass-lined tankers and conveyed to the processing depots. Here it is pasteurized or otherwise processed before being delivered to the consumer. After delivery, care must be taken in the storage and handling of milk and milk bottles.

1. The milk bottle should be kept unopened in a cool larder or preferably a refrigerator, until required.
2. Milk jugs in use should be covered with muslin to keep out dust and flies. They should not be dried with a tea towel, but should be rinsed with boiling water, after washing thoroughly, and drained. Empty milk jugs should be kept in a refrigerator, where possible, to avoid contamination by dust or flies.
3. Milk absorbs smells very quickly. It must be kept apart from strong-smelling foods.
4. Bottles, where still in use, should be rinsed with cold water as soon as emptied, to check the growth of bacteria and to avoid attracting flies. They must not be used for any other purpose and should be returned to the dairy as soon as possible.

Tuberculin-tested milk is produced from herds which are tested for tuberculosis, at frequent intervals, by a veterinary surgeon.

Pasteurized milk is held at a temperature of 71.7 °C (161 °F) for fifteen seconds then rapidly cooled to 4.5 °C (40 °F). This method kills most bacteria without destroying the vitamin content.

Sterilized milk is heated to 100 °C (212 °F) for ten minutes, after which special tests are taken. The cream is well mixed into the milk and does not settle at the top.

Condensed milk. The water is drawn off by evaporation and vitamins added.

Skimmed condensed milk is that from which most of the cream has been removed and is unsuitable for feeding infants.

Dried milk is commonly used as a baby food, the water is drawn off, leaving a fine white powder. The various brands of modified milks available have a list of contents displayed on the packet.

Diseases carried by milk include tuberculosis, typhoid fever, paratyphoid fever, scarlet fever, diphtheria, septic sore throat and undulant fever.

The digestive system

In order to understand what happens to food after it is taken into the mouth, and how it is used by the body for building and repairing tissues, we must know the organs of digestion and how solid foodstuffs are broken down and reduced to a liquid consistency, so that nourishment can be passed directly into the bloodstream to be taken round the body (Fig. 10.1).

The alimentary canal

This is the muscular channel through which all food passes, leading from the mouth to the anus, and lined throughout its length with mucous membrane. The secreted mucus assists the passage of food along the channel.

The alimentary canal is made up of the following.
1. The mouth, with the teeth, the tongue and the salivary glands.
2. The pharynx.
3. The oesophagus or food pipe.
4. The stomach.
5. The duodenum, and the small intestine.
6. The large intestine terminating in the rectum and the anus.

The mouth
The mouth is formed by the lips and the cheeks in front, the hard

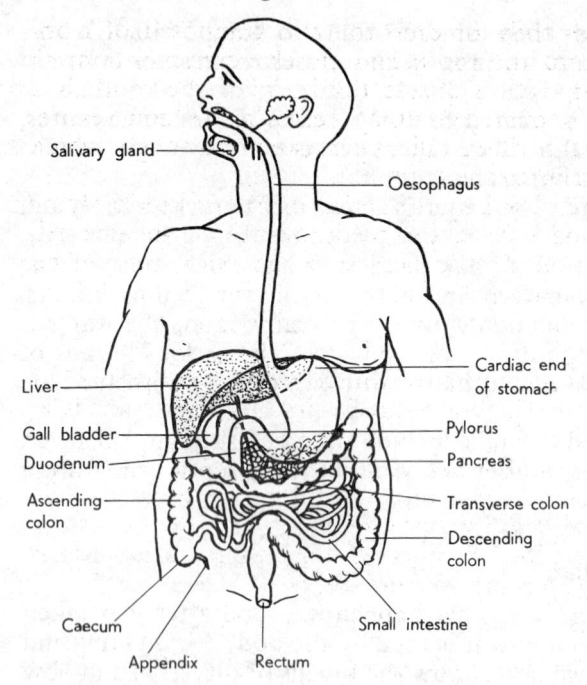

Fig. 10.1 The digestive system.

palate above and the tongue below. The soft palate, or pharynx, lies behind the hard palate in the roof of the mouth.

The teeth
The teeth assist digestion by grinding food so that it is easily dealt with when it enters the stomach. There are two sets, primary and secondary teeth.

Primary teeth are 20 in number, consisting of 8 incisors, 4 canines and 8 molars. This set of teeth is usually complete at 2 to 3 years of age and begins to fall out at 6 to 7 years. By the fourteenth year all the secondary teeth have appeared with the exception of the last four molars, or wisdom teeth, which may appear any time up to the twenty-fifth year.

Permanent teeth number 32; 8 incisors, 4 canines, 8 premolars and 12 molars.

Tooth structure The part of the tooth above the gum is covered with enamel and is known as the crown. The root has one or more fangs covered with cement and is embedded in the bone of the jaw; where the crown and the root meet is the neck

Food, diets and digestion 95

of the tooth. The body of each tooth is composed of ivory which gives shape to the tooth and closely resembles bone in structure and composition. Inside the body of the tooth is a cavity filled with a pulp containing nerves and blood vessels. The tooth socket is lined with periosteum through which nourishment is carried to the teeth.

Decay is brought about by the action of bacteria multiplying on particles of food left on the teeth, destroying the enamel, causing inflammation of the nerves in the pulp cavity, and giving rise to toothache.

The salivary glands
The salivary glands secrete saliva which begins the digestion of starches in the food. There are three pairs of salivary glands in the mouth (Fig. 10.2).
   1. The *parotid glands*, below and slightly in front of the ears.
   2. The *submaxillary glands* under the angles of the lower jaw.
   3. The *sublingual glands* under the tongue.

Salivary ducts are the channels through which saliva passes from the salivary glands into the mouth.

The tongue
The tongue is a muscular organ forming part of the floor of the mouth and is attached to the inside of the lower jaw in front and to the hyoid bone at the back of the mouth. It is the organ of taste and assists in the mastication and swallowing of food.

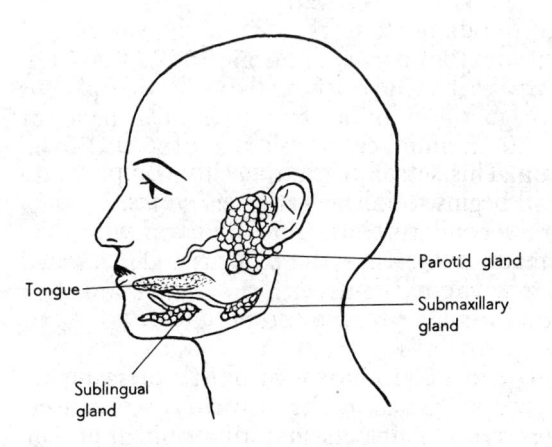

Fig. 10.2 Position of salivary glands.

The pharynx

The pharynx is a muscular cavity lined with mucous membrane, situated between the posterior edge of the soft palate and the epiglottis of the larynx. Below the soft palate it is known as the *oral pharynx*, which passes behind the larynx to join with the oesophagus. That part of the pharynx situated *above* the level of the soft palate is known as the *nasopharynx*. This forms a cavity, lined with ciliated epithelium, into which the posterior nasal cavities open. On the lateral walls are openings of the Eustachian tubes which connect the nasopharynx with the middle ears. At the back of the nasopharynx are two small masses of lymphoid tissue, one on each side. When these become enlarged they are commonly referred to as adenoids. In the act of swallowing, the walls of the pharynx contract, closing the entrances to the larynx, the nostrils and the Eustachian tubes, and passing food back into the oesophagus on its way to the stomach.

The oesophagus

The oesophagus is a muscular tube, 22-25 cm (9-10 in) long, situated behind the trachea, in the neck. It passes through the thorax and pierces the diaphragm to join with the cardiac end of the stomach. The muscle wall of the oesophagus contracts in a wave-like movement to force food downwards into the stomach.

The stomach

The stomach (Fig. 10.3) is an oval, muscular bag lying immediately beneath the diaphragm in front of the spleen and the pancreas. The broad upper part is known as the cardiac end, because it is nearest the heart. The opening from the oesophagus into the stomach is guarded by a strong, circular band of muscle, called the *cardiac sphincter*, which prevents food from rising out of the stomach back into the oesophagus. The only time this may happen is when the stomach wall contracts violently and the sphincter is forced open, as in vomiting. The lower end of the stomach is known as the pylorus and is guarded by the *pyloric sphincter* where it joins with the duodenum. This sphincter prevents food passing through too rapidly.

The stomach wall consists of four coats.

1. An outer serous coat continuous with the peritoneum.
2. A muscular coat consisting of three layers of muscle fibres. Each of these layers contracts in a different direction, longitudinal, circular, and oblique, thus providing a continuous

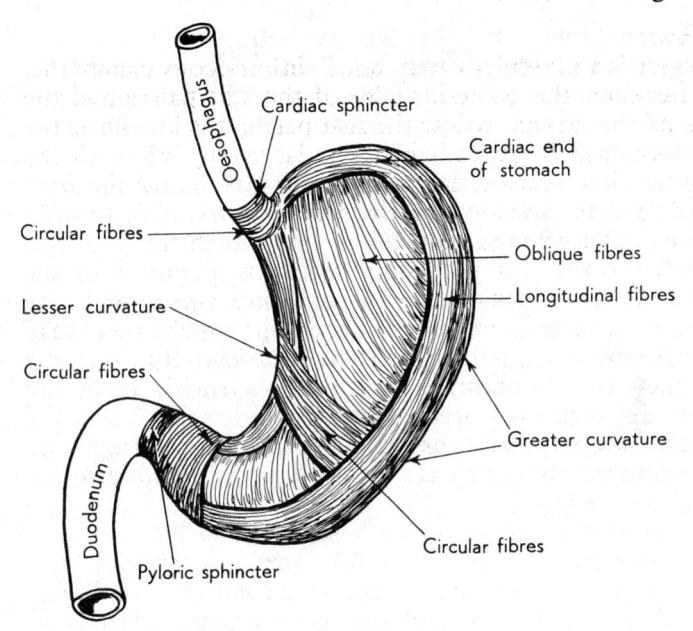

Fig. 10.3 The stomach.

churning movement in all directions, which breaks down and softens the food so that it is readily acted upon by the digestive juices.

3. A submucous coat carrying the blood supply to the walls of the stomach.

4. The inner mucous coat forms the lining of the stomach and secretes mucus. This membrane is drawn up into folds, allowing for distension of the stomach when full, and contains numbers of glands which secrete gastric juices.

The duodenum
The duodenum is the first part of the small intestine and is shaped like a horseshoe, into which the head of the pancreas fits. The duodenum contains a small opening through which digestive juices from the pancreas and the bile from the gallbladder are poured.

The small intestine
The small intestine is about 6.5 m (21-22 ft) long and lies coiled

in the abdominal cavity, held in place by peritoneum.

The upper two-fifths of the small intestine is called the *jejunum*, and the lower three-fifths the *ileum*. The small intestine consists of the same four coats as the stomach, but the muscular coat has no oblique fibres.

The lining of mucous membrane is drawn up into folds and its entire surface covered with fine, hair-like processes called *villi*, giving a velvety appearance.

The walls of the villi are composed of single cells, which allow fluid nourishment to pass through into tiny blood and lymph vessels contained in each of the villi. From these vessels the nourishment is carried into the bloodstream. The mucous membrane lining the intestines is also supplied with numerous glands secreting digestive juices.

Food is passed along the intestines by a continuous wave of muscular contraction and relaxation, known as *peristalsis*.

The large intestine
The large intestine is joined to the small intestine at the ileocaecal valve. The ileum is the last part of the small intestine. The caecum is the beginning of the large intestine. The large intestine is about 1.5 m (5 ft) in length and is divided into the following parts.
1. The caecum.
2. The ascending colon.
3. The transverse colon.
4. The descending colon.
5. The sigmoid colon.
6. The rectum and the anus.

The *caecum* is the blind end at the beginning of the ascending colon and to which is attached the appendix, a tiny, closed tube which sometimes becomes inflamed, causing appendicitis.

The large intestine passes upwards on the right side of the abdomen as the *ascending colon*, turns below the liver, and crosses the front of the abdomen as the *transverse colon*. Under the spleen it turns again to become the *descending colon* on the left side of the abdomen. In the pelvic cavity the large intestine curves to form an S-bend known as the *sigmoid* colon ending in the *rectum*, a muscular tube about 15 cm (6 in) long. The rectum is guarded by a sphincter at the anus, the external opening of the alimentary canal.

The pancreas
The pancreas (see Fig. 10.5) is a gland about 12-13 cm long,

Food, diets and digestion 99

lying behind the stomach. The right end, or head, of the pancreas lies within the curve of the duodenum. The left end, or tail, touches the spleen. Two secretions are formed in the pancreas.
  1. *Pancreatic juice* which aids digestion of food and is poured into the duodenum by the *pancreatic duct.*
  2. *Insulin* secreted by the special sets of cells in the pancreas, known as the islets of Langerhans. Insulin helps in maintaining the correct balance and usage of sugar in the body.

The liver
The liver (Fig. 10.4) is situated immediately under the diaphragm on the right side of the abdomen. It is the largest gland in the body and is divided into two lobes, each consisting of many minute cells. Every one of these liver cells is surrounded by a network of tiny blood vessels, carrying blood rich in nourishment. The blood is collected from the stomach, spleen, pancreas and the intestines and taken to the liver by the *portal vein.*

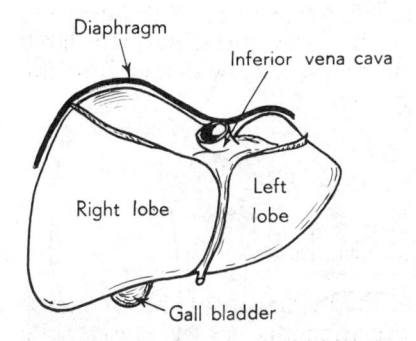

Fig. 10.4 The liver.

  Arterial blood carrying oxygen is supplied to the liver by the *hepatic artery.* The *hepatic vein* carries impure blood away from the liver and empties it into the inferior vena cava.
  Bile is manufactured by liver cells and poured into the *hepatic duct.* This is a canal joining with the cystic duct from the gallbladder, to form the *common bile duct* which opens into the duodenum at the same point as the pancreatic duct.

Functions of the liver
  1. Secretes bile which aids the digestion and absorption of fats.

2. Stores sugar as glycogen until needed by the body.
3. Changes the waste products of protein digestion into urea to be excreted by the kidneys.
4. Manufactures a substance called heparin which prevents the clotting of blood inside the body.

The gall bladder

The gall bladder is a pear-shaped organ in which bile is stored. It is lodged on the under surface of the liver, and connected to it by the cystic duct. When the duodenum is empty, the sphincter guarding the bile duct remains closed. During digestion the sphincter opens to allow bile to be poured into the duodenum (Fig. 10.5).

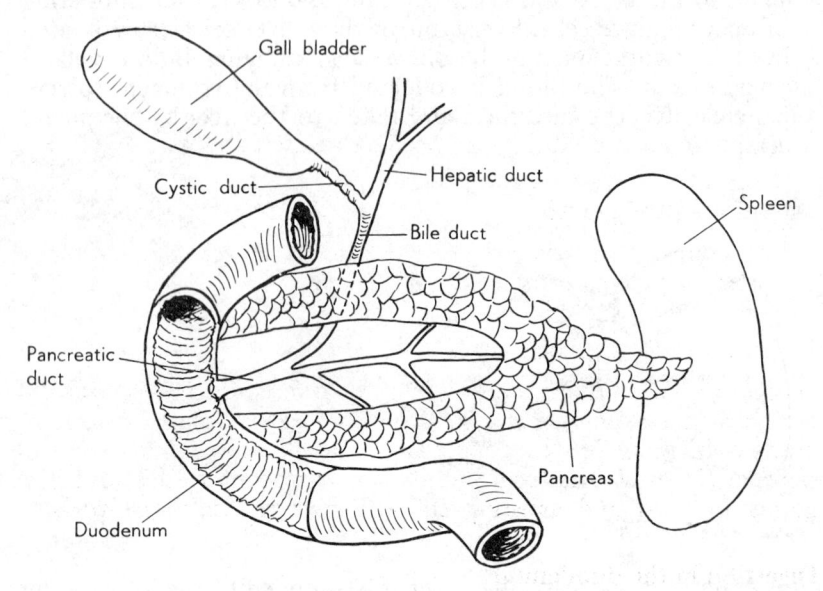

Fig. 10.5 The gall bladder, spleen and pancreas.

The peritoneum

The peritoneum is a double fold of smooth, serous membrane which lines the abdominal cavity, covers some of the abdominal organs, keeping them in place, stores fat which helps to maintain warmth in the body, and secretes a fluid which acts as a lubricant, preventing friction between the constantly moving organs of the abdomen.

Where infection of any of the abdominal organs occurs, the peritoneum becomes attached to the inflamed area in an effort to prevent the infection from spreading. Should perforation of an organ occur, the peritoneum becomes infected, resulting in a serious condition known as peritonitis.

The digestive process

Digestive juices are secreted by various glands in the digestive system. These juices contain chemical substances known as enzymes, which act on food, breaking it down and reducing it to liquid, so that it is easily absorbed by the body tissues.

The digestive process is controlled by the nervous system. Pain, emotion or unpleasant sights or sounds will prevent the secretion of digestive juices and the patient will suffer. On the other hand, contentment and cheerful surroundings will aid the digestion of food and give a feeling of well being. It can be seen that the effect of food served attractively in a pleasant atmosphere is invaluable to the welfare of the patient.

Digestion in the mouth

Saliva contains an enzyme called *ptyalin* which begins the digestion of cooked starches.

Digestion in the stomach

Gastric juice contains *pepsin, rennin* and *hydrochloric acid*.

Pepsin starts the digestion of proteins. *Rennin* turns milk into curds (which are proteins), so that it may be acted upon by the pepsin. *Hydrochloric acid* acts as a disinfectant, destroying germs in food and assisting the enzymes to do their work.

Digestion in the duodenum

Bile and pancreatic juice are poured into the duodenum to continue the digestive process.

Bile breaks down fats and aids peristalsis.

Pancreatic juice contains three enzymes.

1. *Trypsin* continues the digestion of proteins into simple substances known as amino acids.

2. *Amylase* continues the digestion of starches (which was started in the mouth), changing them into simple sugars.

3. *Lipase*, together with bile, acts on fats reducing them to fatty acids and glycerol.

Digestion in the intestines

Other glands continue the digestive process in the intestines, where food is absorbed and waste products removed from the body.

Feeding the patient

Diet is an important factor in the care of the patient. In the first instance it may be ordered by the doctor, but the choice of food is often left to the discretion of the nursing staff. The type and amount of food needed for building and repairing body tissues will depend on the conditon of the patient. It is therefore essential that the nurse should know and understand the individual needs of each patient in her care. Mealtimes are often the highlight of the patient's day, a welcome break in the monotony of ward routine, and should be made as enjoyable as possible.

No treatment should be carried out immediately before a meal is due. All patients should be made comfortable and the ward should be neat, tidy and well ventilated, without draught. Trays, linen, cutlery, silver and glassware should be immaculate and condiment sets clean and well filled.

Attention should be given to the preparation and serving of food. Cold foods should be really cold and served on cold dishes. Hot foods should be taken, on hot plates, to the patient as soon as served. Nothing is more unattractive than the sight of a cold sweet melting on a hot dish or of hot gravy congealing on a cold plate. Servings should be made small and attractive, a plate piled high with food with destroy all desire to eat. A second helping can always be offered where desired. The menu should be as varied as possible, especially for those patients having special diets, which tend to become monotonous owing to the unavoidable limitation of foods allowed. Care must be taken that the correct foods are served to such patients and note should be made of the reaction to food and the amount taken at each meal. Plenty of time should be allowed for the meal, and dishes or plates from the first course removed before the second course is served.

Feeding helpless patients

Few patients enjoy being fed by another person and sometimes, on the slightest provocation, will refuse the food offered. But nourishment is of the utmost importance, on which progress and recovery may rest, and the skilful nurse will ensure that the diet is taken with as much pleasure as possible on the part of the patient. Successful feeding depends to a large extent on the ability and the attitude of the nurse, who, however busy, should show no sign of hurry or impatience. The patient must be given sufficient time to chew and swallow the food without undue haste. Such a meal should not be given in complete silence, but should be accompanied, where possible, by the occasional cheery, non-committal remark which will help to relieve any sense of embarrassment or tension the patient may feel.

The patient should be made comfortable before the food is taken to the bedside, and a table napkin placed under the chin to protect the clothing and bedding. Where solid or semi-solid food is to be given, it should be cut into small pieces. This should not be done at the bedside, but in the kitchen where it may be kept hot during preparation. In transit from the kitchen to the ward, the food should be covered and carried on a tray.

If the patient is nursed in such a position that the food on the plate cannot be seen, an explanation of what is being served should be given with a warning if the food is very hot. A spoon rather than a fork should be used.

For feeding a patient in a recumbent position with fluids a feeding cup with a spout may be used. This type of feeder must be immaculately clean and the spout must be inspected by the nurse before being taken to the patient. To feed the patient, the left arm of the nurse is passed under the pillows and the head slightly raised. The feeding cup is held in the right hand and the fluid allowed to run slowly, one mouthful at a time. The patient may be instructed to control the flow by blocking the spout of the feeding cup with the tongue.

Where a spoon is used for giving fluids, care must be taken that the flow is directed into the side of the mouth. If poured directly over the tongue on to the back of the throat, there is a danger that the patient will cough or choke.

Fluids may also be taken through a straw.

When the feed is finished the mouth is wiped clean with the table napkin and all used crockery removed from the bedside and washed in hot water. Particular attention must be paid to the spout and the angles inside the feeding cup.

Ice to suck is allowed only for some patients. Small pieces of ice are placed on muslin or gauze stretched and tied over the top of a teacup standing in a saucer. Water from the melting ice

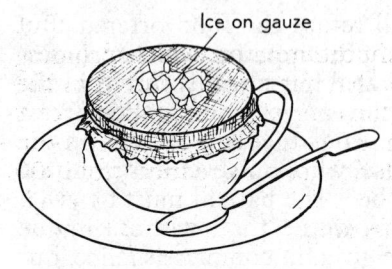

Fig. 10.6 Ice cup.

drips into the cup leaving the dry ice on top. A spoon kept on the saucer is used for handling the ice (Fig. 10.6).

Diets

Full or normal diet is given to patients with good appetites who are on the way to recovery. Such a diet will contain all the necessary food factors in well-balanced proportions.

Light diet is given where the full diet is not easily digested or where bulky meals would be detrimental to the progress of the patient. This diet will contain such foods as steamed white fish, chicken, minced meat, milk and egg puddings and jellies. Extra fluids may be added to the light diet.

Fluid diet consists of nourishing fluids, the basis of which is often milk, which may be flavoured to taste. Soups, fruit juices and eggs beaten in milk may also be given to tempt the patient.

Special diets

Special diets are based on the calorific value of foods. A calorie is a unit of heat, and is a means of judging how much fuel the body needs for the work it has to do. The calorie used in dietetics is a kilocalorie and should be written **kcal** or **Calorie** The new unit now being introduced is the kilojoule (kJ), 4.2 kJ = 1 kcal.

The average calorific requirements for healthy adults are as follows.
Manual workers doing heavy work   4000 calories per day.
Moderately heavy workers   3000-3500 calories per day.
Sedentary workers   2500-3000 calories per day.
Women usually need fewer calories than men.

Where food is taken in excess of the calorific needs of the body, it will be laid down as fat.

Food, diets and digestion

Reducing diet
A reducing diet is devised to satisfy the appetite whilst excluding those foods which make fat, so that fat already stored in the body can be utilized to provide the energy required. Where it is necessary for reasons of health to reduce the weight, as in diabetes or gross obesity, the calories may be reduced to 1000 per day.

The following foods are not fattening.

Salads without oil or dressing.

Clear soups.

Fresh or stewed fruit without sugar.

Green vegetables such as sprouts, cabbage, French beans, cauliflower, spinach, leeks, lettuce, marrow, swedes or turnips.

Forbidden foods are sweets, sugars, chocolate, jams, marmalade, and honey.

Dates, nuts, raisins, preserved, dried and tinned fruits.

Starches in the form of breads, cakes, flour in any form, puddings or sweet biscuits.

Fats such as dripping, lard, suet, bacon, olive oil or mayonnaise.

Drinks not to be taken include beers and bottled drinks of all kinds, especially fruit squashes.

Patients on a reducing diet should be weighed each week at the same time and in the same clothes. The weight should be recorded on the chart. Visitors should be advised against bringing articles of food for any patient on a special diet.

A high calorie diet is designed to increase weight, especially after severe illness. Extra carbohydrates, fats, milk, and glucose are added to the normal diet.

A low protein diet is used for patients suffering from nephritis (inflammation of the kidney) or from uraemia. Plenty of sugar, fruit and vegetables are given. Proteins are restricted to lessen the work of the kidneys.

A high protein diet is given where repair of the body tissues is essential, as in severe burns, or chronic or subacute nephritis.

Low fat diet. Fats are reduced to a minimum where there is jaundice due to inflammation of the gall bladder (cholecystitis).

Low salt or salt-free diet. This may be ordered where gross oedema is present, as in congestive heart failure or hypertension (high blood pressure). No table salt is allowed and no salt used in cooking. Forbidden foods include salt fish or meat, bacon, chocolate and foods containing baking powder or bicarbonate of soda.

A low residue diet contains no roughage and is designed to reduce peristaltic action (see p. 98). This diet is given to patients suffering from inflammation or ulceration of the colon (colitis) or from diarrhoea. It is a bland, non-irritating diet, commencing with diluted milk and milk foods and progressing to sieved vegetables and fruit pulp. Skins and pips of fruits must be avoided.

Gastric diet. In the treatment of gastric and duodenal disorders, diet plays an extremely important part. The object is to provide sufficient nourishment without stimulating the secretion of gastric juice. To avoid this, small quantities of bland, non-irritating foods are given frequently to prevent the stomach from becoming empty. The basis of the diet consists of milk with eggs, butter, strained orange juice, minced white meats, white fish and sieved vegetables. In the early stages, milk is given at two hourly intervals. Other foods are added gradually as the patient progresses.

Diabetic diet. The consumption of sugars and carbohydrates is controlled. The diet varies according to the age and weight of the patient and the stage of the disease, and is compiled by the dietitian on the instruction of the physician.

When meals are being served it is the responsibility of the nurse to ensure that the right diet is given to the right patient. If a mistake *is* made, the patient on a special diet will usually accept what appears to be a welcome change of foods and will rarely question what is served, but the wrong diet may have serious consequences. A nurse who is in any doubt should not hesitate to ask for guidance from the ward sister or nurse in charge.

Disorders of the digestive system

Dyspepsia

Dyspepsia, or indigestion, is due to various factors concerned with eating habits, e.g. failure to chew food sufficiently, consistently hurried meals, eating undigestible foods such as hot bread, rich pastry or unripe fruit and over-eating. Lack of exercise and constipation may also cause dyspepsia.

Symptoms are discomfort or pain in the region of the stomach, flatulence, nausea, vomiting and heartburn. (Heartburn is a burning sensation in the chest caused by the acid gastric juice rising into the oesophagus).

Treatment

The cause of the dyspepsia is traced and the remedy found. This is usually sufficient to alleviate the symptoms. A light diet taken in small amounts may be advised. Fluids should not be taken with meals as this tends to dilute the gastric juice.

Peptic ulcer

Peptic ulcer is ulceration of the mucous membrane of those parts of the stomach or duodenum which are in contact with the gastric juice. Medical treatment includes complete rest in bed, freedom from worry, and a bland non-irritating diet. Antacids such as magnesium trisilicate may be ordered to lessen the acidity in the stomach. A special diet consisting of frequent small milk feeds is given. Where medical treatment is not successful, the ulcerated portion of the stomach or duodenum may be removed by operation.

Life for the gastric patient is very trying and often made miserable by pain and discomfort. The treatment is long and tedious, and the constant emphasis on food and its effect often results in dissatisfaction and irritability. The nurse caring for such a patient must show the utmost patience and tolerance and should remain calm and cheerful at all times. Everything possible should be done for the patient's mental and physical comfort. Drinks and meals should be served promptly. The patient should not be kept waiting. Mouth hygiene should be carried out before and after each feed, especially if the patient is on a milk diet.

Pyloric stenosis

Pyloric stenosis may occur in the newly born. The pyloric sphincter of the stomach is so constricted that food cannot pass through. The condition does not become evident until the third or fourth week of life when the baby cries a great deal, appears very hungry and does not gain weight, although taking feeds. Projectile vomiting occurs, i.e. the contents of the stomach are thrown for some distance. Early operation is usually necessary and the fibres of the pyloric sphincter are divided to enlarge the opening.

Cholecystitis

Cholecystitis is inflammation of the gall bladder. *Gall-stones* may form in the gall bladder and may vary in size. Sometimes a gall-stone will obstruct the common bile duct causing acute pain, jaundice and collapse. Removal of the gall bladder is known as *cholecystectomy*.

Jaundice

Jaundice is the yellow discoloration of the skin and conjuctiva of the eyes, owing to the presence of bile pigment in the blood. In cholecystitis, jaundice is often accompanied by putty-coloured stools (see p. 28).

Enteritis

Enteritis is inflammation of the small or large intestine and may be due to bacterial infection or to food poisoning.

Gastroenteritis

Gastroenteritis is a dangerous infectious disease and every case should be isolated. Extreme care must be taken when dealing with soiled linen and stools (see p. 129). Disposable napkins should be used for infants. Hospital policy with regard to disposal of infected linen and disposables must be strictly adhered to. The chief symptoms are severe diarrhoea and vomiting, hyperpyrexia, loss of weight, exhaustion and collapse. The disease progresses rapidly and collapse may occur within twenty-four to forty-eight hours.

Nursing care

The patient must be kept warm. This often entails constant watching where the bed-clothes are repeatedly thrown off.

Tepid sponging may be ordered to reduce the hyperpyrexia. Fluids only are given as prescribed. In severe cases nothing is given by mouth and the patient has fluids given intravenously to rest the gastrointestinal tract. The amount of fluids taken and the number of stools must be strictly recorded on the fluid chart. A mouth tray should be kept at the bedside and the mouth cleansed at frequent intervals. Pressure areas must be treated four-hourly, or more often where necessary.

The nurse must take every possible precaution against the spread of the disease, because gastroenteritis is extremely infectious and its effect may be disastrous, especially where children and infants are concerned.

Artificial feeding

Where food cannot be taken by mouth in the usual way, as during unconsciousness, shock or disease causing paralysis or obstruction of some part of the upper digestive tract, the patient is artifically fed. This may be done via a nasogastric tube or via a gastrostomy tube.

General principles of artificial feeding

Feeds given should contain the maximum amount of nourishment. Protein, carbohydrates (especially sugar), vitamins and mineral salts should be included in the fluid diet. Milk, clear soups, egg flip and any strained foods which will pass through the catheters can be given. Feeds should be prepared at a temperature of 38 °C (100 °F). Strict oral hygiene must be observed in all patients who are not eating normally, to keep the mouth moist.

Requirements.
 1. For passing nasogastric tube.
 Tray containing
 Prepacked nasogastric tube of appropriate size.
 Spigot.
 Ten-ml or 20-ml syringe.
 Blue litmus paper.
 Strapping.
 Vomit bowl and cover.
 Box of mediwipes or cotton-wool balls.
 Gallipot with warm water.
 Receptacle for soiled articles.

 2. For administering feed.
 Measure containing feed standing in a bowl of warm water.
 Thermometer.
 Funnel, tubing, connection, spring clip.
 Sixty-ml measure containing cooled, boiled water or fresh drinking water.
 Serviette.

Method
The forthcoming procedure is explained to the patient and the bed screened. If possible, the patient is nursed in the sitting position, well supported by pillows. Tissues are offered so that the patient may blow his nose. If this is not possible, the nurse

should cleanse the nostrils with pledgets of cotton wool.

A tissue is placed around the neck and the tip of the tube moistened in warm water. The tube is then passed gently into one nostril. To assist passage of the tube, the patient is asked to keep swallowing and to resist coughing if possible. If severe coughing, retching or cyanosis occur, the tube is slightly withdrawn and the patient reassured before continuing. Stomach contents are aspirated and tested on the litmus paper. Acid stomach contents will turn blue litmus paper red. The tube is now secured out of the line of vision with strapping, and the spigot inserted until feeding is commenced. The tube is normally left in situ for subsequent feeds.

To begin feeding, the temperature of the feed is checked and should be 38 °C. Air is expelled from the funnel and tubing by filling with water and attaching the spring clip. The funnel and tubing are attached to the nasogastric tube by means of a connection and the feed is given slowly. The funnel must not empty or air will enter the stomach causing discomfort. At the end of the feed a little water is passed down the tube to rinse it and, after disconnection of the funnel and tubing, the nasogastric tube is spigotted. The feed is recorded and the patient left comfortable. The apparatus is thoroughly washed and rinsed and either kept for a subsequent feed or changed for a fresh pack, according to hospital policy.

Gastrostomy feeding

This method is adopted where there is obstruction of the oesophagus and no food can be taken by mouth. An artificial opening is made into the stomach through the abdominal wall and a self-retaining catheter inserted, which is closed with a spigot. Through this tube the patient is fed with liquid foods containing the maximum amount of nourishment. Feeds are given as ordered, usually every two to four hours during the first forty-eight hours after operation and increased gradually. The area round the wound must be well protected with a sterile, oily dressing in case there is leakage of gastric juice on to the skin of the abdomen causing severe soreness.

The requirements are as for nasogastric feeding (see p. 109), with the addition of protection for the bedding.

Method
The patient should be placed in the position found to be most comfortable and the bed-clothes folded down over the lower abdomen.

Food, diets and digestion

The protective towel is arranged to protect the dressing. All air must be expelled from the tubing before commencing the feed by running a little sterile water through. The spigot is removed from the abdominal tube and the feeding apparatus connected to it. Thirty millilitres of the water are run through first. (If this produces pain or discomfort, it may be an indication that the fluid is entering the peritoneal cavity. Should this occur, the feed is stopped and the nurse in charge informed). The sterile water is followed by the feed, which should be given very slowly. When the feed is finished, the second 30 ml of water is run in to ensure that the gastric tube is clear of obstruction. Should the tube become blocked, a little solution of bicarbonate of soda should be run in.

A gastrostomy dressing is usually arranged in such a manner that it need not be disturbed during feeding, but should the dressing require renewal it must be done with strict aseptic precautions. Frequent mouth hygiene must be carried out, because no food or drink can be taken by mouth, and sores may result from neglect in this manner (see p. 39). Where the gastrostomy is permanent, the patient is taught how to self-administer the feeds, together with instruction on the hygiene of the skin round the wound and cleaning of equipment.

11
The lymphatic system

The lymphatic system consists of lymphatic capillaries and larger vessels, lymphatic glands and ducts, all of which conduct the lymphatic fluid towards the thorax. These vessels are provided with valves allowing lymph to pass in one direction only. Lymph is a clear, watery fluid, similar in composition to blood plasma, and containing mineral salts and cells called lymphocytes, which are similar to white blood cells. Lymph comes from the blood and is forced through capillary walls to surround and bathe the tissues in fluid and assist in removing waste matter. Excess lymph, not needed by the tissues, is collected by the lymphatic vessels and poured back into the bloodstream at the root of the neck where the internal jugular veins join with the subclavian veins. Lymphatic vessels from the right side of the head, neck and right arm and the right side of the thorax join to form the *right lymphatic duct* which returns the lymph to the bloodstream at the *right side* of the neck. Lymph from the rest of the body is collected into the *thoracic duct*, situated in the chest, and poured into the bloodstream at the *left* side of the neck (Fig. 11.1).

Lymphatic glands have a beaded appearance and are found in groups in many parts of the body. As the lymph passes through the glands it is filtered so that bacteria are prevented from entering the bloodstream. Lymphocytes are produced in the lymphatic glands.

Functions of the lymphatic system

1. Transport and filtration of lymph.
2. Destruction of micro-organisms and phagocytes.
3. Formation of lymphocytes.
4. Formation of antibodies and antitoxins.

The lymphatic system 113

Shaded area indicates lymph collected by the right lymphatic duct

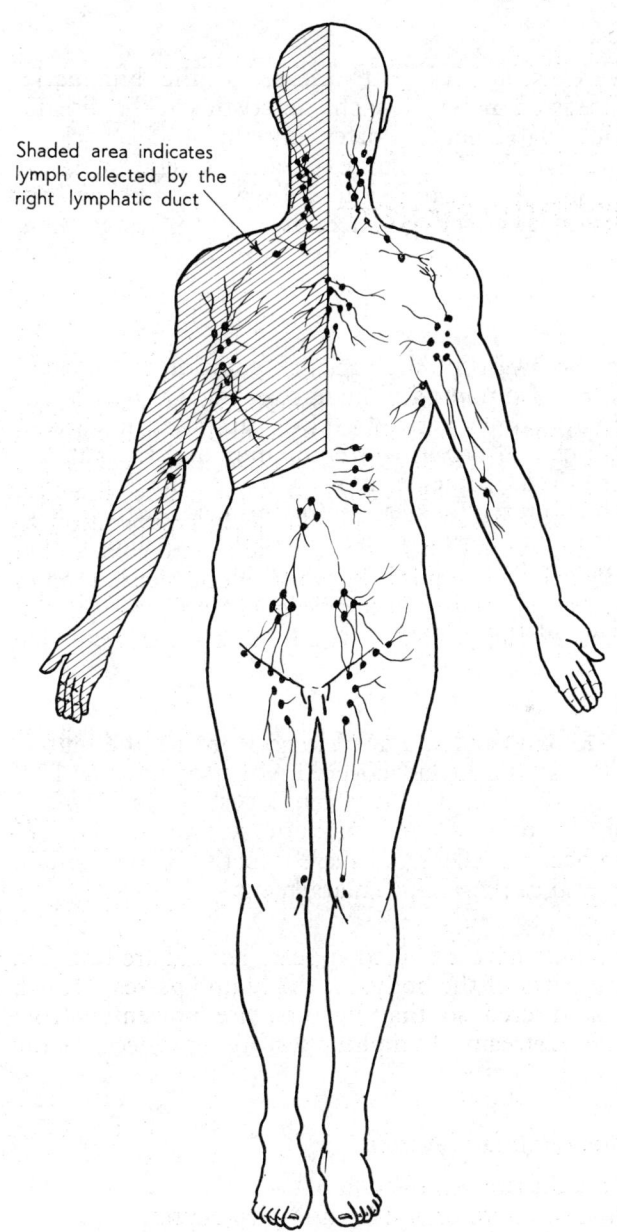

Fig. 11.1 The lymphatic system.

Hodgkin's disease

Hodgkin's disease is a malignant disease of the lymphatic system. The cause is unknown. The characteristics of the disease are lymph node enlargement — often initially in the neck — accompanied by weight loss, pyrexia and general malaise.

Treatment is usually a combination of drugs and radiotherapy and the prognosis, although guarded, is slightly better than previously.

Nursing care

The nurse must be aware of the patient's emotional state and needs to give a lot of support and understanding. Current treatment, although sometimes very effective, can have unpleasant side effects. Nausea and vomiting are common and the patient usually feels very tired. Anti-emetics may be prescribed, and the patient should be tempted by small, frequent meals, attractively served. Strict attention must be paid to oral toilet and, if the patient is confined to bed, regular turning and pressure area care are important in the prevention of bedsores. These patients are often very thin and debilitated.

The spleen

The spleen, 12-13 cm (about 5½ in) long, is in the abdominal cavity behind the stomach and covered with peritoneum. The spleen is closely allied to the lymphatic system and, where enlargement of any part of the lymphatic system occurs, the spleen may also become enlarged. Severe infective diseases, such as malaria, may also cause splenic enlargement.

12
The endocrine glands

Endocrine glands are situated in various parts of the body and secrete chemical substances, known as hormones, which are passed directly into the bloodstream. Any alteration in the normal amount of a hormone produced may have a serious effect on the body. The most important endocrine glands (Fig. 12.1) are as follows.
　1. The pituitary gland situated at the base of the brain.
　2. The thyroid gland in the front of the neck.
　3. The four parathyroid glands lying behind the thyroid gland.
　4. The thymus gland behind the sternum.
　5. The suprarenal or adrenal glands, one on the upper surface of each kidney.
　6. The pancreas behind the stomach.
　7. The gonads or sex glands.

The pituitary glands

The pituitary gland is known as the master gland because it governs the activity of all other endocrine glands. It is divided into the anterior and posterior lobes, each of which secrete hormones having important work to do in the body. The anterior lobe produces a hormone which controls growth, especially of bone. In childhood, deficiency of this hormone causes dwarfism and oversecretion causes the bones of the skeleton to become greatly enlarged, a condition called *gigantism*. In adults, oversecretion results in overgrowth of the bones of the hands, feet and face, a condition known as *acromegaly*. Other hormones secreted by the anterior lobe of the pituitary gland influence the reproductive organs and the activity of the thyroid gland and stimulate part of the suprarenal glands to produce cortisone.
　The posterior lobe of the pituitary gland produces hormones which cause the contraction of the involuntary muscles of the

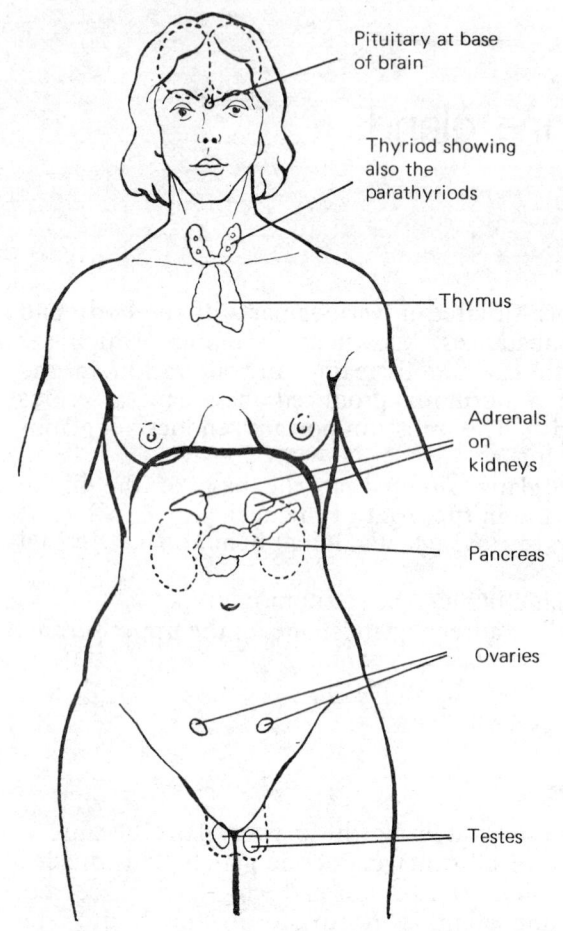

Fig. 12.1 The endocrine glands.

bladder, intestines and uterus, and raise the blood pressure. One hormone also influences the secretion of urine by the kidneys.

The thyroid gland

The thyroid gland consists of two lobes, one on each side of the larynx, joined by a central, narrow strip known as the isthmus (Fig. 12.2). The thyroid gland produces the hormone *thyroxine* which is essential for normal growth and mental development. Deficiency of this hormone in childhood causes *cretinism*, a

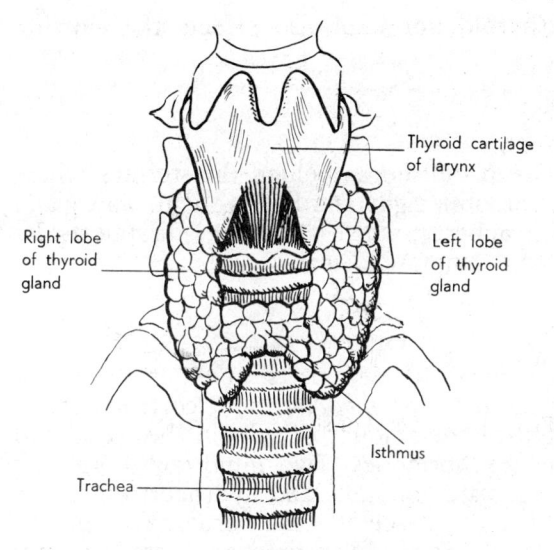

Fig. 12.2 The thyroid gland.

condition in which physical growth is retarded and the child is mentally subnormal. In the adult, lack of this hormone results in *myxoedema*, marked by thickening of the skin, puffiness of the face, falling hair, lethargy and slowness of speech. Treatment with thyroid extract may be ordered for the relief of these symptoms. Enlargement of the thyroid gland and oversecretion of thyroxine give rise to *Grave's disease* or *thyrotoxicosis*. The chief signs and symptoms are nervousness, irritability, loss of weight (although the patient may have a good appetite), sweating, rapid pulse and staring eyes. Such patients may be treated medically or surgically, but in all cases they should be kept quiet. Noise, excitement and worry should be avoided and the patient reassured in times of stress.

The parathyroid glands

The parathyroid glands are four small glands lying behind the thyroid gland, two on either side. They produce a hormone which controls the balance of calcium in the blood and the amount of calcium deposited in bone. Lack of this hormone causes *tetany*, a condition in which the muscles go into spasms, particularly those of the hands and feet (carpopedal spasm). The muscles of the jaw may be affected, especially when touched. The parathyroid hormone also affects the clotting power of the blood.

The thymus gland

The thymus gland lies in the thorax behind the sternum where the trachea divides into the right and left bronchi. This gland increases in size until puberty, when it gradually disappears. Its function is thought to be immunological.

The adrenal glands

The adrenal glands consist of two parts, the outer part, or *cortex*, and the inner part, or *medulla*. The cortex secretes hormones which control the amount of salts in the blood and the secretion of the sex hormones. Two important hormones produced by the cortex are cortisone and hydrocortisone. The medulla of the adrenal glands secretes the hormone adrenaline which prepares the body for action in times of stress or danger by increasing the heart beat, raising the blood pressure and causing the liver to release more glucose for use by the muscles. Adrenaline has the same effect as the sympathetic nervous system (p. 160). Addison's disease is the result of failure of the adrenal glands to function efficiently, and is commonly treated with hydrocortisione. The nursing care is as for any severe illness.

The islets of Langerhans

The islets of Langerhans are special cells scattered throughout the *pancreas*. They secrete insulin which controls the balance of sugar in the blood. An insufficiency of insulin leads to diabetes mellitus.

The sex glands

The sex glands include the ovaries in the female and the testes in the male. The ovaries secrete two hormones, oestrogen and progesterone, which have an effect on the menstrual cycle and reproduction. The testes produce the hormone testosterone which is also concerned with reproduction.

13

Administration of medicines

The prescription of drugs is the duty of the doctor, but it is the nurse's responsibility to see that they are given.

Legislation

The Misuse of Drugs Act 1971

All drugs controlled by this Act are termed controlled drugs. They include morphine, diamorphine and pethidine as well as the amphetamines and others.

These drugs are kept in a separate cupboard marked C.D. and the key is kept by the ward sister or her deputy. A record of each dose administered is kept in the Controlled Drugs Register. Hospital practice may vary, but usually two nurses, one of whom is a registered nurse, check and administer these drugs.

The Medicines Act 1968

Most other drugs used in hospitals come under this Act. They are stored in a different, locked cupboard.

Administration of medicines

Medicines may be given by the following routes.
   1. By mouth in the form of liquids, pills, tablets, capsules or powders.
    2. By inhalation.
    3. By inunction i.e. rubbing into the skin.
    4. By injection − intramuscular, hypodermic, intravenous.
    5. Rectally in the form of a suppository or as an enema.
    6. Topically − eye, ear or nose drops or ointments.

120 *Practical nursing*

Prescription sheets

These may vary slightly from hospital to hospital, but follow a common pattern.

The prescription sheet must state clearly:
1. name, age and hospital number of patient;
2. the *approved* name of the drug;
3. the dose in metric units;
4. the date of the prescription;
5. the route by which the drug is to be given;
6. the times at which the drug is to be given.

A doctor's signature must accompany each prescription. Regular prescriptions have a column for the signature of the nurse administering the medicine.

'Once only' prescriptions appear on a separate section of the sheet to avoid confusion.

No drug must be given to a patient in hospital without the written prescription of a doctor.

Oral medicines

Requirements
1. Lockable trolley containing all necessary medicines.
2. Bowl of warm soapy water.
3. Medicine measures and medicine spoons.
4. Saucers or trays.
5. Tissues.
6. Jug of water or fruit juice (or use patients' own individual jugs).

Method
At the patient's bedside.
1. Read the prescription sheet carefully.
2. Select medicine and read label — check with prescription.
3. Read checking column to ensure medicine has not already been given.
4. Invert bottle several times holding a finger over the top.
5. Unscrew top and lay it, inner surface up, on trolley.
6. Hold measure at eye level and pour prescribed amount, keeping bottle label uppermost.
7. Replace the top on the bottle and put the medicine on the saucer or tray.
8. Check the patient's name band with the prescription sheet.

Administration of medicines

9. Give the medicine to the patient and remain at the bedside until it is swallowed.
10. Offer water or fruit juice.
11. Record the administration on the prescription sheet.

After the medicine round has been completed, all bottles should be wiped clean before being stored in the cupboard.

Tablets or capsules
Steps 1 to 3 as above.
4. Tip the required number into a spoon and place this on a saucer or tray.
5. Replace the bottle top.
6. Check the patient's name band with the prescription sheet.
7. Give the tablet with a glass of water and ensure that it is swallowed.
8. Record the administration on the prescription sheet.

Suppositories or enemas
The same rules for checking apply.
For requirements see pages 29 and 30.

Intramuscular injections

These injections are given deep into a muscle, usually in the front or outer aspect of the thigh or into the buttocks. The site of the injection must be carefully chosen because there is great danger of the needle piercing a vein, a nerve or the periosteum of a bone. This is particularly important when giving an injection into the buttocks, to avoid damage to the sciatic nerve. A cross should be marked on the buttock with the finger and the injection given into the upper and outer quarter, well away from the centre of the cross (Fig. 13.1).

Requirements
Tray with:
    Syringe — usually 2 ml;
    No. 1 (dark green) needle;
    mediswabs;
    drug;
    ampoule of water for injection, if required;
    file, if necessary;
    prescription sheet.

122 *Practical nursing*

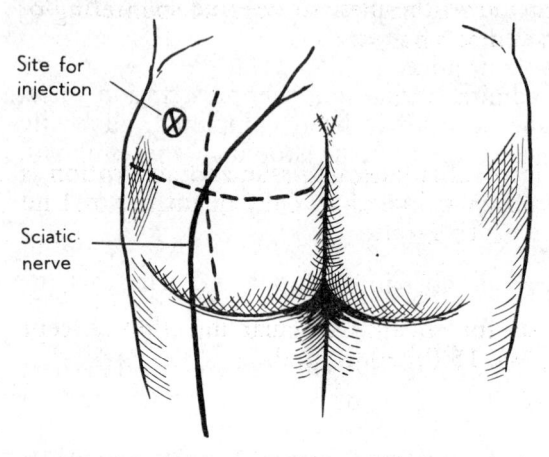

Fig. 13.1 Site for intramuscular injection.

Method
The hands should be thoroughly washed and a strict aseptic technique used. The syringe is attached to the needle, which should remain in its plastic sheath. If a vial with a rubber diaphragm is used, this is cleaned with a mediswab and, once the needle has pierced the diaphragm, a small quantity of air is injected to facilitate removal of the contents. The required amount is drawn into the syringe, and the syringe held at eye-level to check the dose. After withdrawal of the needle, the plastic sheath is replaced to maintain sterility. The tray and prescription sheet are taken to the bedside and the procedure is explained to the patient. Screens should be drawn to maintain privacy.

When giving an intramuscular injection, the syringe is held at right angles to the skin and the needle inserted deep into the muscle. Before injecting the drug, the plunger of the syringe should be withdrawn slightly to make sure that the needle has not punctured a vein. The injection should be given slowly and, after removing the needle, the area should be gently massaged with a swab to encourage the absorption of the drug.

When preparing injections, particularly antibiotics, care must be taken not to spill any of the drug on the hands.

When using glass ampoules, the contents are shaken below the neck and the top snapped off. Most ampoules do not require the use of a file, but care is needed to prevent splintering of glass and injury to the nurse's hands.

Hypodermic injections

These are injections into subcutaneous tissue and absorption is slower than by intramuscular injection. Only quantities of 1 ml or less should be given via this route.

Requirements.
These are the same as for an intramuscular injection, except that a smaller needle, No. 15 (blue), is used.

Method
The preparation is as described above for intramuscular injection.
　　Explain to the patient what is to be done. Clean the skin over the site of the injection with the mediswab. Take up a fold of skin free of veins with the thumb and forefinger and quickly insert the needle in a slightly upward direction.
　　An alternative method is to stretch the skin over the site of the injection with the thumb and forefinger before swiftly inserting the needle. This is often less painful than the above method and is particularly useful in obese patients where a fold of skin is somewhat difficult to grasp. For either method, the syringe should lie almost flat against the skin.
　　Release the skin and slowly push in the piston.
　　Place a mediswab over the puncture before withdrawing the needle, then gently massage the area to ensure distribution of the drug.

Intravenous injections

These are given by a doctor, but the nurse may be responsible for their preparation.

Requirements
These are as for intramuscular injections.
　　In addition a rubber tourniquet may be required if an intravenous infusion is not in progress.
　　The doctor must check the dose of the drug and the vial before administration of the injection.

124 Practical nursing

Intravenous infusions

Requirements
- Prescribed intravenous fluid.
- Infusion stand.
- Recipient set.
- Assortment of cannulae.
- Adhesive strapping.
- Splint, if necessary, for limb.
- Mediswabs.
- Tourniquet.
- Waterproof to protect bed.
- Fluid balance chart.

In addition
- Equipment for shaving area, if necessary.
- Anglepoise lamp.

Method
After checking, the bag of prescribed fluid is hung from the infusion stand and the needle of the recipient set inserted into the appropriate part after removal of the protective cap. The control is opened to allow fluid to run down the recipient set, thus expelling air. When this is achieved, the protected end is kept covered until the doctor has performed the venepuncture. Once attached to the cannula, the rate is regulated carefully and strapping at the site of the venepuncture completed according to the doctor's wishes. The fluid balance chart is filled up with the appropriate details.

After the procedure, the patient is made comfortable and his locker put within reach of his free hand. The fingers should be checked regularly for colour and temperature and swelling, and the site of the infusion must also be checked for signs of swelling or infection.

Classification of drugs

General anaesthetics, such as nitrous oxide, produce complete loss of consciousness.

Local anaesthetics produce loss of feeling in the area to which they are applied, e.g. cocaine, procaine and novocaine.

Analgesics are drugs which relieve pain, e.g. morphine, pethidine, aspirin and codeine.

Antibiotics are substances prepared from certain living

Administration of medicines 125

moulds and fungi. They prevent the growth and multiplication of harmful bacteria. Examples are penicillin, erythromycin and aureomycin.

Anticoagulants are substances which prevent blood from clotting inside the body, e.g. Heparin or Dindevan in coronary or venous thrombosis.

Antidotes are used to counteract the effect of poisons.

Aperients are drugs such as Bisacodyl and senna, which produce action of the bowels.

Diuretics are given to increase the output of urine by their action on the kidneys. Examples are frusemide and chlorothiazide.

Emetics are substances which induce vomiting and include salt in water, or mustard in water and Ipecacuanha. Apart from the latter, which is used in paediatrics, emetics are rarely employed. Gastric lavage is usually safer if it is necessary to empty the stomach.

Expectorants are drugs which stimulate the coughing-up of mucus from the lungs.

Hypnotics are those drugs which induce sleep and have no effect on pain, e.g. chloral hydrate and the barbiturates. Examples of barbiturates are Soneryl, Nembutal and Amytal.

Narcotics produce deep sleep during which pain is not felt. Examples are Morphine, Omnopon and Pethidine.

Sedatives are drugs which lessen excitement and reduce activity, but do not always induce sleep.

Tranquillizers are used for the relief of anxiety and disturbed mental states and include diazepam and chlorpromazine.

14
Micro-organisms and infection

Micro-organisms, such as bacteria, are of animal or vegetable origin and may be divided into those which are harmless to man and those causing disease. These latter, for continued existence, may need warmth, food, moisture and darkness. All these conditions are to be found in the body, and after invading living tissue, the harmful bacteria multiply and produce toxins which give rise to disease. Extreme heat or cold will kill them although some are very difficult to destroy.

The chief varieties of disease-carrying micro-organisms are as follows.
1. Cocci.
2. Bacilli.
3. Viruses.
4. Spirochaetes.
5. Fungi.
6. Protozoa.

Bacteria

1 *Cocci* are rounded organisms of several types which, under the microscope, are seen to grow in different formations.

(*a*) *Staphylococci* may cause septic skin lesions such as carbuncles or impetigo, or more serious conditions such as meningitis, disease of the middle ear or septicaemia.

Staphylococci are numerous on the surface of healthy skin, especially round the fingernails. It is, therefore, most important that the nurse should keep the hands and nails scrupulously clean to prevent the spread of infection by staphylococci.

(*b*) *Streptococci* may cause such diseases as acute tonsillitis, scarlet fever, impetigo or pneumonia.

(*c*) *Pneumococci* cause pneumonia and conditions of acute inflammation with pus.

(*d*) *Meningococci* give rise to inflammation of the meninges (see p. 159).
(*e*) *Gonococci* cause venereal disease with inflammation of some part of the reproductive system.

2. *Bacilli* are rod-shaped organisms giving rise to serious diseases such as tuberculosis, diphtheria, tetanus, whooping cough, food poisoning or dysentery.

3. *Viruses* are micro-organisms too small to be seen under the light microscope and are difficult to isolate and control. They are the cause of measles, German measles, influenza, the common cold, poliomyelitis, mumps, chicken-pox and smallpox.

4. *Spirochaetes* are larger than either cocci or bacilli. The outstanding infectious disease caused by spirochaetes is the venereal disease, syphilis.

5. *Fungi* are vegetable parasites which attack hair, skin or nails, causing ringworm or infecting the mucous membrane of the mouth, causing thrush.

6. *Protozoa* are animal organisms which give rise to malaria, sleeping sickness and amoebic dysentery.

Aspects of infectious diseases

Harmful bacteria may enter the body by three common routes.
1. By their inhalation with air into the respiratory system.
2. By ingestion, i.e. taking of infected food or fluid by mouth.
3. By inoculation, where such organisms enter through a break in the skin or mucous membrane, caused by injury or the bite of an insect.

Spread of infection

An infectious disease is one which is passed directly or indirectly from one person to another and may be spread in the following ways.

1. *Direct contact* with a patient suffering from infectious disease, as by kissing or contamination of the skin by discharges from the body of the infected person.

2. *Indirect contact*. Infection may be carried by the following.

(*a*) *Fomites,* which is the name given to all articles handled by the patient and includes books, toys, handkerchiefs, crockery, etc.

(*b*) *Airborne infection* may occur as *droplet* infection. Bacteria and viruses are spread in droplets of moisture expelled from the nose or mouth during careless coughing or sneezing.

(c) *Dustborne organisms* are carried in dust. Germs from excretions, such as sputum, are released to float into the air and become a source of danger to other people.

3. *Carriers* may be human, animal, or insect.

(a) *Human carriers* are people who carry the disease-causing organisms in the body tissues and pass them on to others, but do not themselves suffer from the disease they carry. They are unaware of the infection they carry and are therefore a source of great danger to the community. During an outbreak of infectious disease, carriers may be difficult to trace, but when identified they are kept in isolation and treated, until declared free from the infecting organism. Gastroenteritis, typhoid and diphtheria may all be spread by human carriers.

(b) *Animal carriers* may carry such diseases as rabies from infected dogs, anthrax from sheep or cattle, or bubonic plague from rats.

(c) *Insect carriers.* The most common insect carrier is the house fly with its unclean habits. Infection is carried on the body and in the excretions of the fly as it travels from animal or human excreta directly to exposed food or feeding utensils. Other insect carriers are the mosquito which spreads malaria and the tsetse-fly which carries sleeping sickness.

Prevention of the spread of infection

Contamination of the food or water supplies may have serious consequences in the community. These services are constantly being supervised by the Public Health Departments of the Local Authorities. These are under the supervision of Medical Officers of Health, who in turn are responsible to the Department of Health for the well being of the population in their areas. Should an outbreak of infectious disease occur, the Medical Officer of Health has the power to close schools or public places where necessary, to stop the sale of food or milk and to isolate any person suspected of having been in contact with, suffering from, or carrying infectious disease. The Medical Officer of Health attempts to prevent the spread of infection in the following ways.

1. Notification.
2. Isolation.
3. Barrier nursing.
4. Immunization.

Notification
By law, certain infectious diseases must be notified by the doctor in charge of the patient, to the Medical Officer of Health of the area in which the patient is living at the time the disease was contracted. In the case of major infectious disease, such as smallpox, diphtheria, typhoid, etc., the staff of the Public Health Departments will endeavour to trace all contacts of the infected person or persons so that they may be quarantined until all danger of further infection is passed.

Isolation
Isolation is the separation of the patient from those not suffering from the disease until all risk of infection is passed.

Barrier nursing
Barrier nursing is carried out during the illness of the patient and is the means of preventing the spread of infection to other people. Every person having contact with the patient must observe certain rules. Gowns and, in certain circumstances, masks must be worn by all personnel entering the room. Damp dusting and vacuuming using a filter should be done to prevent infected dust from rising into the air.

All articles used by the patient, including crockery, cutlery, and toilet articles must be kept separately, clearly marked with the name of the patient and sterilized immediately after use. As many items as possible should be disposable.

Charts, notes, report forms, x-rays and other documents should be kept outside the patient's room.

All linen and disposable items are sealed in plastic bags and disposed of according to hospital policy.

In severe gastrointestinal infection faeces or other contaminated excreta may have to be covered with a disinfectant for an hour prior to disposal. Group or hospital disinfection policy should be followed.

On recovery, various tests are carried out to determine whether the patient is free from infection. When this has been proved, terminal disinfection is carried out.

Terminal disinfection All disposable equipment is put in appropriate receptacles for burning.

All linen, used or unused, is sent to the laundry, following the local procedures for infected linen.

Non-disposable items are soaked in disinfectant or preferably sterilized.

Furniture, walls and floor are washed with hot water and detergent and left for twenty-four hours before reuse.

If infection has been severe, formaldehyde gas may be used to disinfect the room and contents. All articles for disinfection are spread out, and doors and windows sealed. When the gas is discharged into the room the door is sealed from the outside. After twelve hours the room can be thoroughly aired and washed in the usual manner.

Immunization

Immunity is the ability of the body to resist infection and may be natural or acquired. When bacteria or viruses enter the body they produce toxins which set in motion the defence mechanism of the blood. White blood cells, or leucocytes, react to the toxins by manufacturing antibodies. These antibodies are substances which, when produced in sufficient quantities, destroy the invading bacteria. Each type of infectious disease produces its own antibodies which will have no effect on any other disease. For example, a child may be immune to measles after an attack of the disease, but not to chicken-pox or diphtheria.

Natural immunity may be inherited. Babies under the age of 6 months are usually immune to common infectious diseases, especially those to which the mothers are immune, but as the child grows older the immunity may be lessened. Many people remain immune to certain types of infection throughout their lives.

Natural acquired immunity may result from overcoming an infectious disease by the manufacture of sufficient antibodies in the body to give complete immunity; or where an individual is exposed to repeated doses of an infection, too small to cause symptoms of the disease, but which stimulate the production of sufficient protective antibodies in the bloodstream to give immunity.

Artificially acquired immunity may be active or passive.

Active artificial immunity is produced by an injection into the body of a vaccine which stimulates the bloodstream to manufacture its own antibodies.

Passive artificial immunity is the use of injections of serum already containing antibodies, so that the blood does not need to make its own. This serum is prepared from the blood of an already immunized animal or from a human who has had the disease and is immune from it. Examples of such sera are the antidiphtheric serum and antitetanus serum.

Serum sickness may follow an injection of serum and may produce severe symptoms such as asthma, urticaria, oedema or hay fever, especially in people who have a tendency towards these disorders. This hazard can now be prevented by the use of human tetanus immunoglobulin for injured patients who are not immunized.

Terms used in relation to infectious disease

1. *Incubation* is the period between the entry of invading bacteria into the body and the appearance of the first signs and symptoms of the disease. During this time the micro-organisms multiply and manufacture toxins which cause illness. The incubation period varies with each disease.

2. *Isolation* is the period during which the infected person is kept apart from other people until clear of the infective organism. This period also varies with each disease.

3. *Quarantine* is the period during which contacts of the infected person are isolated. This is usually the incubation period plus an extra few days.

Outbreaks of infectious disease are spoken of in the following terms.

1. Sporadic: isolated cases appearing in scattered areas.
2. Epidemic: the incidence of many cases in one area, at the same time.
3. Pandemic means worldwide; the disease spreads all over the world.
4. Endemic diseases are those which constantly arise in particular areas of the world, e.g. malaria, found in swampy areas.

Infectious diseases

Chicken-pox

The incubation period is fourteen to twenty-one days. Chicken-pox is a mild infectious disease caused by a virus and usually spread by direct contact or by infected articles. All age groups may be affected, the first sign being an irritating rash over the face, trunk and limbs. Efforts should be made to discourage scratching to avoid infection and permanent scarring of the skin. Isolation is necessary until all crusts have disappeared.

Measles

The incubation period is ten to fourteen days. This is a virus infection spread by droplet infection. It is most infectious before the appearance of the rash and is especially dangerous in children under 5 years of age. The condition starts with all the signs of a heavy cold, accompanied by a hard dry cough and red, watering eyes. About the second day, small white spots appear inside the cheeks. These are known as Koplik's spots and are an important sign of measles. On the fourth day the rash appears behind the ears, spreading over the face and neck, and the temperature rises. The child should be kept warm in bed in a well-ventilated room. If the eyes are very sore, they should be bathed twice a day and no reading allowed. The room should be shaded from bright light. Where the cough is distressing, a steam inhalation will bring relief. The diet should be light with plenty of fluids and frequent mouth washes given between meals.

Complications of measles may be earache (otitis), bronchopneumonia, gastroenteritis or thrush. Strict watch should be kept for any signs of pain in the ear and respiratory difficulties, or gastric disturbances. In the later stages of the disease a high protein diet should be given.

German measles

The incubation period is fourteen to twenty-one days. This is also a virus infection, spread by droplet infection. Few symptoms appear but there may be headache, malaise or swelling of the lymphatic glands in the neck. The rash appears on the first or second day after which all symptoms, including the rash, may disappear. The patient must be kept in isolation, although no special nursing care is needed and complications are rare. The main importance of this disease is the fact that, if occuring during the first three or four months of pregnancy, there is risk that the unborn child will suffer from some serious defect. Active immunization with rubella vaccine is offered to all girls at puberty. **Under no circumstances** should pregnant women, or those who may become pregnant during the following eight weeks, be given the vaccine.

Mumps

The incubation period is twelve to twenty-six days. This is a highly infectious disease caused by a virus and spread by droplet infection. The main symptoms are swelling of the lymphatic glands in the neck, and the parotid gland in front of the ear, cauisng pain in the face and neck. The temperature rises, but falls as the swelling subsides. The face should be kept warm, using kaolin poultices and cotton-wool pads if the pain is severe. The diet should consist of soft, bland foods which will not stimulate the secretion of saliva by the glands, with plenty of fluids. Fruits and acid sweets should be avoided. It is most important that the mouth should be kept clean with frequent mouth washes.

Complications arise when other glands in the body become affected. In the female the breasts or ovaries may be affected and in the male the testes may become inflamed, giving rise to orchitis. Encephalitis is also a rare complication.

Whooping cough

The incubation period is seven to fourteen days. It is caused by a bacillus and spread by droplet infection. The disease usually attacks children, although adults who are not immune may also be affected.

The first signs are those of a heavy cold and catarrh, with a rise in temperature. This stage lasts about one week. The cough follows during the second or third week and is known as the paroxysmal stage. Violent attacks of coughing occur, during which the child may hold the breath and become cyanosed, ending in a long, deep noisy inspiration called the 'whoop'. Vomiting may follow a bout of coughing and in severe cases the child should be fed after each attack to avoid malnutrition. This stage may last for several weeks, the bouts of coughing being more frequent at night. The child should be kept in a warm, well-ventilated room, although not necessarily in bed, and should be kept quietly occupied.

The diet should be light and nourishing.

Complications are convulsions in the very young, bronchitis or bronchopneumonia, and more rarely hernia or prolapse of the rectum.

The mortality rate is highest during the first years of life. Vaccination against whooping cough may be obtained and is usually combined with antidiphtheria and antitetanus vaccine, given during the first months of life.

Scarlet fever

The incubation period is one to seven days. This is due to streptococcal infection and is spread by droplets, by contaminated foods, particularly milk, and more rarely by carriers. The onset is sudden with rapid pulse, headache, sore throat, pyrexia, shivering, vomiting and swollen glands in the neck. The tongue is furred and appears to be covered with bright red spots, referred to as 'strawberry tongue'. The face is flushed with an area of pallor round the mouth. The rash appears on the second day on the neck and chest, later spreading all over the body. This fades in about six days, after which the skin peels off, a process known as desquamation. The patient must be isolated. While the throat is sore and the temperature high, the diet should consist mainly of fluids. Tepid sponging should be carried out to help reduce a high temperature, gargles given for the sore throat and kaolin poultices applied to the neck where pain from the swollen glands is severe.

Complications are otitis media, bronchitis, pneumonia, acute nephritis, inflammation of the coats of the heart, arthritis or rheumatism.

Diphtheria.

The incubation period is two to seven days. It is spread by direct contact, by droplet infection, by carriers, by infected articles and in milk. The disease has been almost eradicated in the United Kingdom since immunization was introduced. However, the danger of infection is always present in children who have not been immunized. Many people do not appreciate this danger and should be encouraged to continue immunization of their children.

The first signs and symptoms are those of a severe toxaemia

and include sore throat, headache, rapid pulse, pallor, swelling of the glands of the neck and a greyish-white membrane forming over the tonsil area. In severe cases this membrane spreads over the larynx and trachea, causing asphyxiation, in which case tracheostomy is carried out to relieve the obstruction.

Complications may include bronchopneumonia, damage to the heart structure or heart failure, albuminuria and paralysis, especially of the soft palate or eye muscles.

The enteric fevers

The enteric fevers — typhoid and paratyphoid — are caused by salmonella organisms. The diseases are spread by the contamination of water, milk or food, usually where there is poor sanitation.

Travellers and others at risk can be immunized with TAB vaccine.

Carriers of the disease put others at risk by contamination of water supplies and food.

Poliomyelitis

The incubation period is considered to be five to fourteen days, but there is a possibility that it may be longer. This disease is caused by a virus infection which attacks nerve structures lying in the anterior, or front portion, of the spinal cord, resulting in paralysis of different groups of muscles. The widespread use of polio vaccine has markedly reduced the incidence of the disease in the United Kingdom.

15
Disinfection and sterilization Surgical nursing

Disinfection

Bacteria need warmth, darkness and dampness in order to grow and multiply. These conditions must be excluded and bacteria destroyed by disinfection and sterilization. Articles to be sterilized must be spotlessly clean or the process will be useless. There are three methods of disinfection by which bacteria are destroyed.

Natural disinfection

Natural disinfection by the ultraviolet rays in sunlight which kill bacteria, and by the action of wind which dries and renders them harmless.

Gamma irradiation

Gamma rays are being increasingly used by industry to sterilize prepacked goods.

Chemical disinfection

Chemical disinfection is achieved by the use of liquid or gaseous agents. Liquid agents are commonly known as disinfectants. Articles to be sterilized by this method must be completely covered with the disinfectant of the correct strength and for the correct time needed for the destruction of germs.

Physical disinfection

Physical disinfection is the use of extreme dry or moist heat.

Dry heat
Burning, of infected articles such as books, papers, toys or toilet particles used by the patient and soiled dressings from the wards.

Baking in specially constructed ovens through which hot air is circulated.

Moist heat
Boiling, by which articles to be sterilized are completely immersed in boiling water and boiled for at least five minutes. Where infection has been severe, boiling must be continued for a longer period. Spores can survive boiling and so this method should only be used if nothing better is available.

Steam under pressure in an *autoclave*. The articles to be sterilized are subjected to steam under pressure for a specified time, then thoroughly dried by vacuum.

Sterilization of equipment

A Central Sterilization Supply Department (CSSD) is now available to most hospitals. Here all equipment needed for sterile procedures is made up into individual packs of disposable materials and sterilized by autoclaving or by gamma radiation or in an infra-red heated tunnel. The staff of the CSSD issue the packs daily to the wards as required. Each pack is sealed with a sensitive strip of paper which changes colour when sterilization is complete. The colour of this strip must be checked by the nurse immediately before use to ensure that the contents are sterile. If there is any doubt as to its sterility or if the pack is torn or damaged in any way it should be discarded and returned to the CSSD.

Ward sterilization of equipment

If equipment is required in an emergency and is not available sterile, chemical disinfection may be used. It must be emphasized that this is a poor substitute for autoclaving.

An alcohol-based disinfectant is normally used and the nurse must follow the group/hospital policy on the matter. Irrespective of the agent used, the following apply.
1. The article must be thoroughly cleaned before immersion. Blood or other contaminants will prevent action of the agent.
2. The disinfectant must be used at the recommended strength.
3. The recommended time of immersion must be strictly adhered to.
4. The article must be completely immersed.

Surgical nursing

Preparation of a patient for operation

Except in emergency, patients for operation are usually admitted to the wards at least one day beforehand. This gives the patient the opportunity to become familiar with hospital routine and the surroundings in which he will be nursed during recovery. Many simple operations are done on a day admission basis. Written consent for the administration of an anaesthetic and for operation must be obtained from the patient and in the case of a child, the consent of the parent or guardian. This is the duty of the doctor who must first explain the nature of the operation to the patient or parent.

Mental preparation
Most people are nervous of undergoing an operation, some are frightened. Nervousness and fear before an operation may have a detrimental effect afterwards, unless reassurance is given.

During the waiting period, the nurse must do everything possible to instil confidence into the patient, being prepared to explain simply the pre-operative routine and the reasons for the various necessary procedures. A calm and cheerful manner will help a great deal to dispel any feeling of apprehension on the part of the patient.

Physical preparation
On the day before operation the skin over the operation area is shaved and the patient has a bath. A specimen of urine is collected and tested for any abnormalities. The results are noted and any abnormality reported. During the preceding night, good restful sleep is essential. If anxiety prevents the patient from sleeping, the night nurse should report the fact. A sedative may be ordered.

Day of operation
A light meal consisting of tea or Bovril and toast is given at least four hours before the time of operation. No food or drink must be given after this.

The patient is then dressed in a theatre gown. Where a female patient has long hair, it should be arranged in two plaits for comfort. Hair pins and grips must be removed. Make-up and nail varnish must be removed.

Disinfection and sterilization Surgical nursing

False teeth are put in the patient's denture box and kept in a safe place.

Rings and ear-rings should be removed and handed to the ward sister for safe keeping.

The bladder should be emptied immediately before the premedication is given.

Great care must be taken to ensure that the correct notes and x-rays are taken to the theatre with the patient. The *first names* as well as the surname of the patient must be checked with those on the notes. The identity label must also be checked with the notes and attached firmly to the wrist or ankle before the patient leaves the ward. This is extremely important to avoid any mistake in identity being made.

Premedication

Certain drugs are given from a half to one hour before the scheduled time of operation. These drugs are written on the patient's prescription sheet by the doctor and usually include atropine or scopolamine to reduce the secretion of mucus in the mouth and respiratory passages, together with a sedative such as morphine or Omnopon. After the premedication has been administered, the patient must be left to rest quietly behind screens but should be kept under observation.

The nurse escorting the patient to the theatre must take the patient's notes and x-rays.

Postoperative care

When the patient has been taken to the operating theatre, the bed is stripped and made up with clean linen. The top clothes are folded into a pack. Instead of pillows, a waterproof protection and pillowslip or anaesthetic towel are placed at the top of the bed.

Oxygen and suction apparatus are available at the bedside and a vomit bowl and cover placed on the locker.

A tray containing the following should also be on hand (Fig. 15.1):

mouth gag;
tongue depressor;
tongue forceps;
sponge-holding forceps;
gauze swabs.

On the return journey from the theatre to the ward, the patient must be warmly covered and must be closely watched

140 Practical nursing

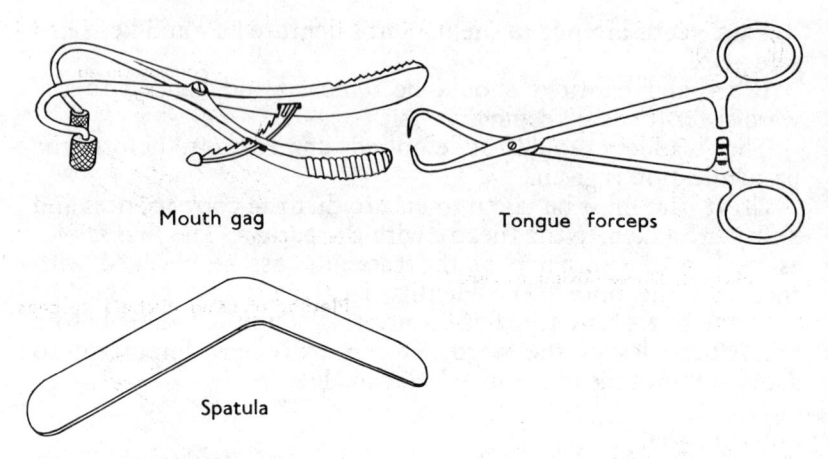

Fig. 15.1 Surgical instruments.

for any signs of coughing, vomiting or blueness of the face. An airway is usually placed in the mouth before the patient leaves the theatre, to prevent obstruction of the air passages, and is left in position until the patient recovers consciousness. The head must be turned to one side as long as the patient remains unconscious. Constant watch must be kept at the bedside until recovery from the anaesthetic.

Observations of temperature, pulse, respirations and blood pressure are made as ordered. Depending on the type of surgery, fluids may be allowed four hours postoperatively, but nothing should be given without specific instructions. Drugs such as pethidine and morphine may be prescribed for pain.

Following sedation and a sleep, the patient should have face and hands washed and be changed into night clothes if the condition permits.

Postoperative urinary retention is not uncommon and the nurse should note when the patient passes urine for the first time.

Ward dressings

In surgical nursing the chief aim is to keep all wounds free from germs which cause inflammation and sepsis.

Disinfection and sterilization Surgical nursing 141

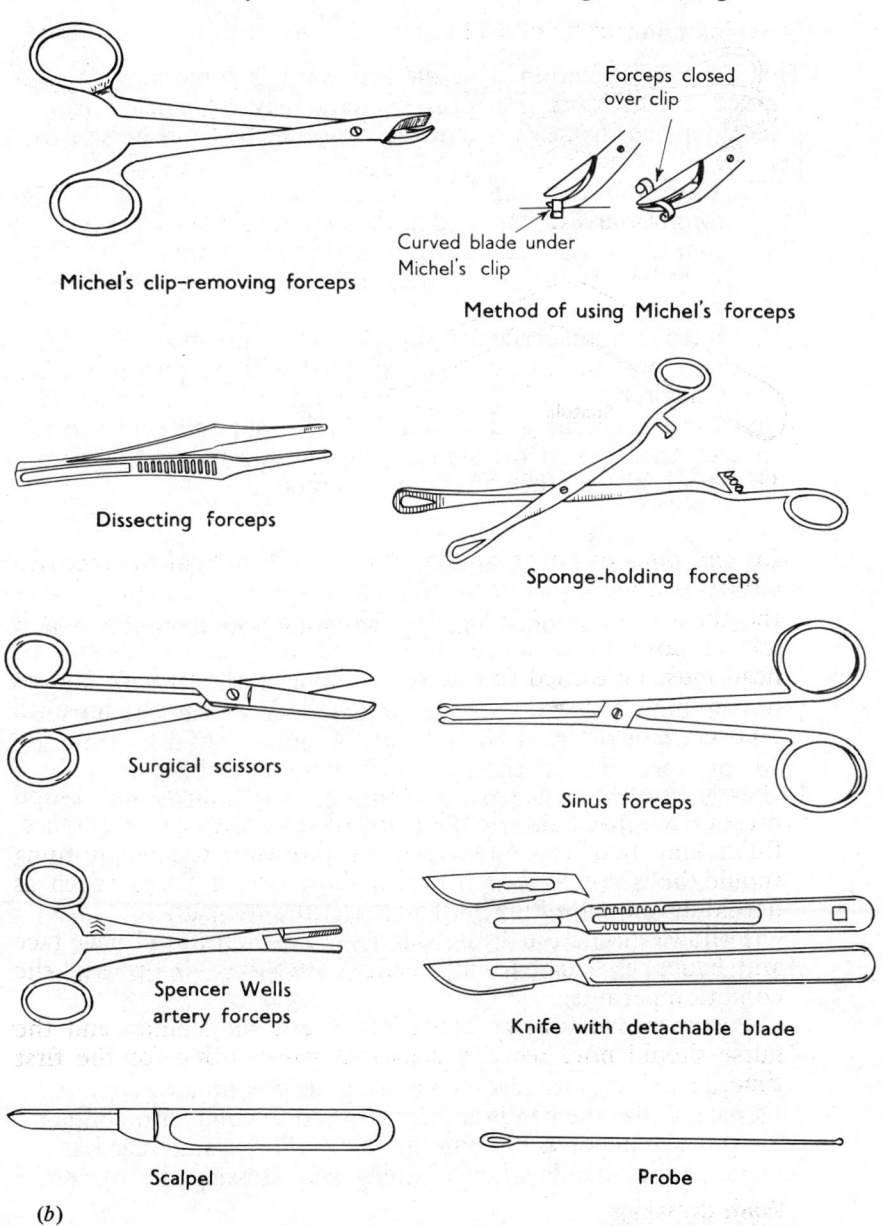

Michel's clip-removing forceps

Forceps closed over clip

Curved blade under Michel's clip

Method of using Michel's forceps

Dissecting forceps

Sponge-holding forceps

Surgical scissors

Sinus forceps

Spencer Wells artery forceps

Knife with detachable blade

Scalpel

Probe

(b)

Fig. 1.b

Cross-infection

This type of infection in a surgical ward is something to be avoided at all costs. Harmful bacteria may be carried from place to place, from one article to another or from person to person.

The chief sources of infection are as follows.
1. From bacteria in dust and in the air.
2. From the noses and mouths of staff and patients.
3. On toilet articles and other equipment in common use in the ward.
4. On trolleys, unsterile dressings and instruments.
5. On hands, which must be regarded with suspicion at all times. Certain bacteria are present on the cleanest skin, especially round the fingernails and cuticles. Nails should be kept short. Cuts and scratches of the skin should be reported to the ward sister before sterile procedures are undertaken.

Prevention of cross-infection

Ward cleaning and bed-making should be completed at least one hour before dressings are commenced. It is better, however, if dressings can be done in a separate room away from the main ward.

To reduce the risk of droplet infection during the dressing, there should be no unnecessary talking either from the nurses at the bedside or from the patient. No nurse suffering from a cold or sore throat should assist with dressings. In some hospitals, masks are worn for dressings, but policies do vary.

Clean wounds are dressed first. Septic wounds last.

No wound must be uncovered until everything is ready for the renewal of the dressing.

Containers holding presterilized packs must never be placed on the floor or they will become contaminated by bacteria in the dust and dirt which will cling to the bases of the packs.

Ward dressing procedure

All sterile dressings are carried out using the *non-touch technique.* This means that the hands are not allowed to come into contact with the wound or the sterile dressings. Forceps are used as a second pair of hands when cleaning and dressing the wound.

Dresser's assistant

The bed is screened and the patient told what is happening. The trolley is taken to the bedside by the assistant, who then prepares the patient. The bedding should be turned down neatly and carefully and the clothing removed as far as is necessary. The patient must be made as comfortable as possible. After washing the hands, the assistant loosens the tape holding the dressing in place.

The dresser
The hands and arms are washed thoroughly in hot water with soap for two minutes, then rinsed and dried on a clean towel. Drying the hands and arms prevents drips of contaminated water from falling on the sterile instruments or into the wound.

The soiled dressing is removed with dressing forceps and put into a disposable paper bag or into a soiled-dressing pedal bin. The forceps are discarded into a second paper bag used for soiled instruments *only*. Sterile towels are placed in position round the wound.

A second, clean pair of forceps is then used to swab the skin round the wound, working away from the incision. This is done so that the bacteria from the surrounding skin are not washed into the wound. The central portion of the incision is cleansed last.

At this point, other instruments, such as sinus forceps, probe, clip-removing forceps or stitch scissors may be required. Each is placed in the bag for soiled instruments when finished with.

Finally, yet another pair of sterile forceps is used to handle the clean dressings covering the wound. The bandage is reapplied, with the help of the assistant, the pillows rearranged and the patient made comfortable.

The trolley is removed and cleared. The necks of the bags containing used instruments or soiled dressings must be tightly twisted and the bags placed in their respective containers for collection. Instruments should be returned to the Central Sterilization Depot and the dirty dressings put into the disposal bins. Unused, clean dressings may be returned for resterilization.

Basic dressing trolley (Fig. 15.2)

The lower shelf carries all unsterile equipment needed and should be prepared first. The top shelf is completely sterile. The hands should be washed before swabbing the trolley and again before the top shelf is prepared. The rails and shelves are washed thoroughly using a swab soaked in spirit or the disinfectant in use in the hospital. Then hands must be washed again at this point and a face mask put on, if necessary. When

144 *Practical nursing*

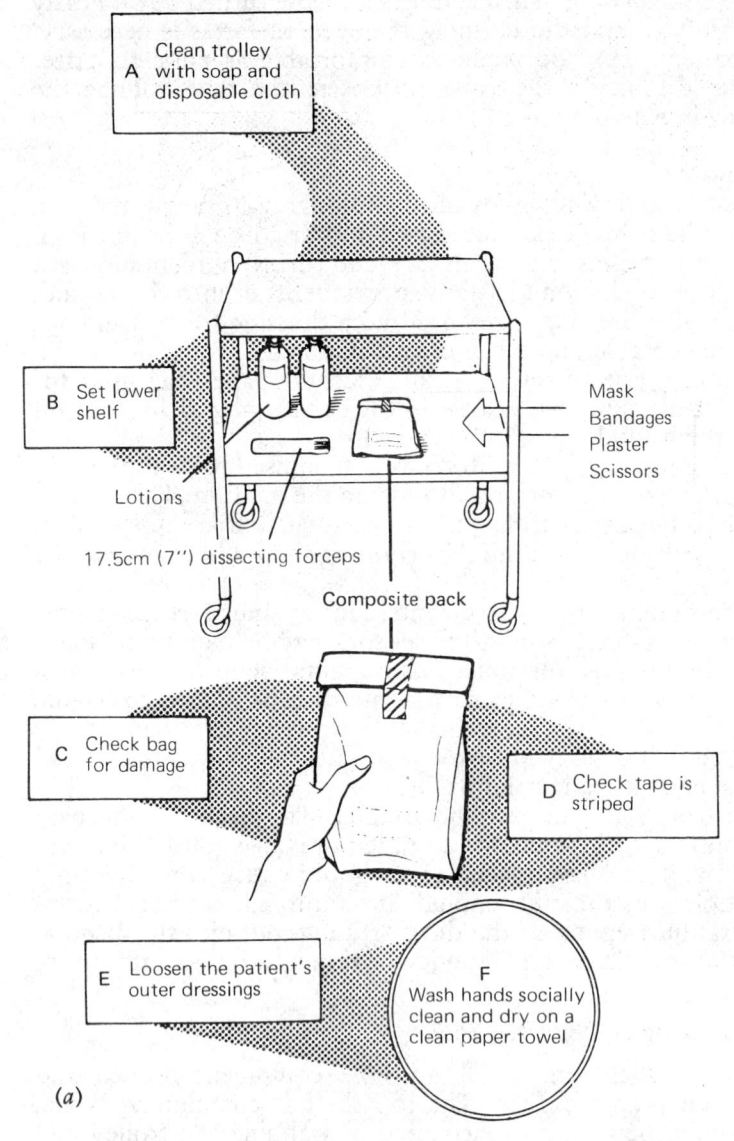

A Clean trolley with soap and disposable cloth

B Set lower shelf

Mask
Bandages
Plaster
Scissors

Lotions

17.5cm (7″) dissecting forceps

Composite pack

C Check bag for damage

D Check tape is striped

E Loosen the patient's outer dressings

F Wash hands socially clean and dry on a clean paper towel

(a)

Fig. 15.2 Ward dressings. (From Sacharin and Hunter. *Paediatric Nursing Procedures.* Livingstone, London.)

Disinfection and sterilization Surgical nursing 145

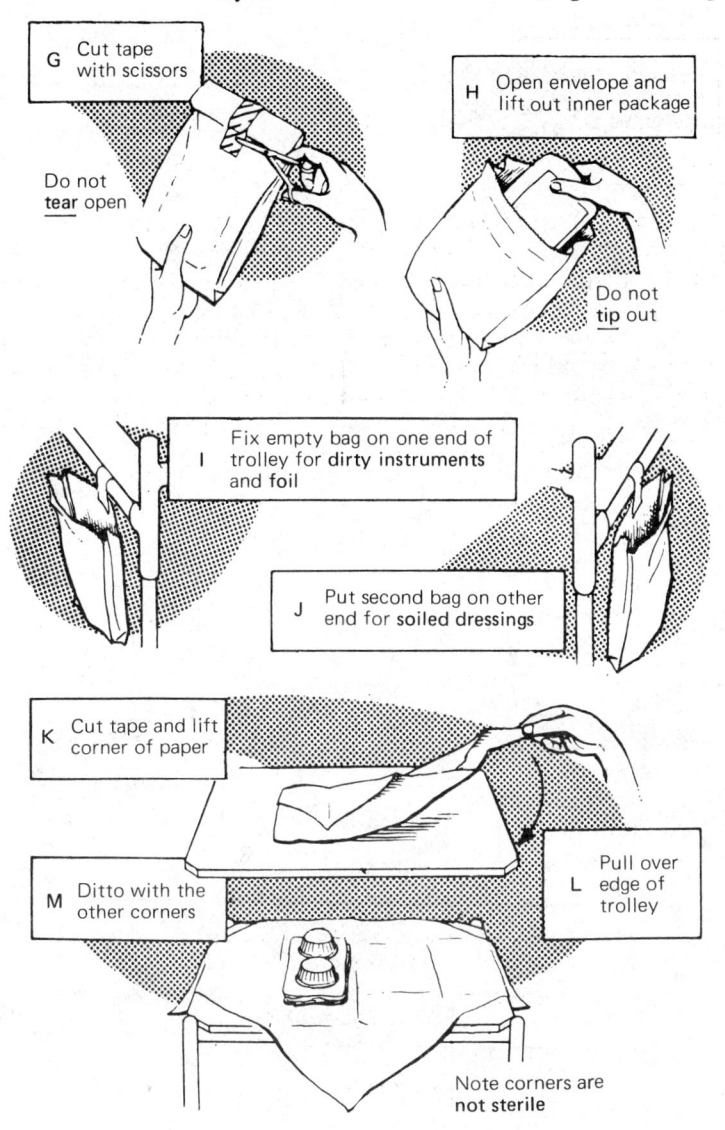

G Cut tape with scissors

Do not **tear** open

H Open envelope and lift out inner package

Do not **tip** out

I Fix empty bag on one end of trolley for **dirty instruments and foil**

J Put second bag on other end for **soiled dressings**

K Cut tape and lift corner of paper

L Pull over edge of trolley

M Ditto with the other corners

Note corners are **not sterile**

Fig. 2.b

146 *Practical nursing*

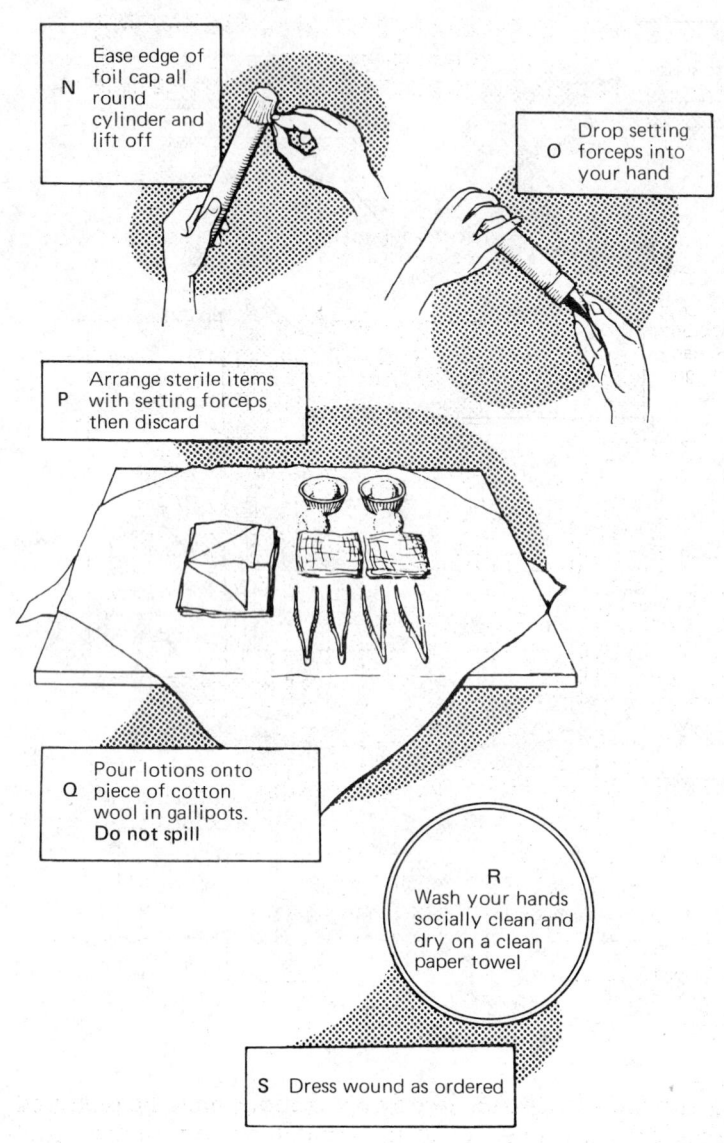

- N Ease edge of foil cap all round cylinder and lift off
- O Drop setting forceps into your hand
- P Arrange sterile items with setting forceps then discard
- Q Pour lotions onto piece of cotton wool in gallipots. **Do not spill**
- R Wash your hands socially clean and dry on a clean paper towel
- S Dress wound as ordered

Fig. 2.c

Disinfection and sterilization Surgical nursing 147

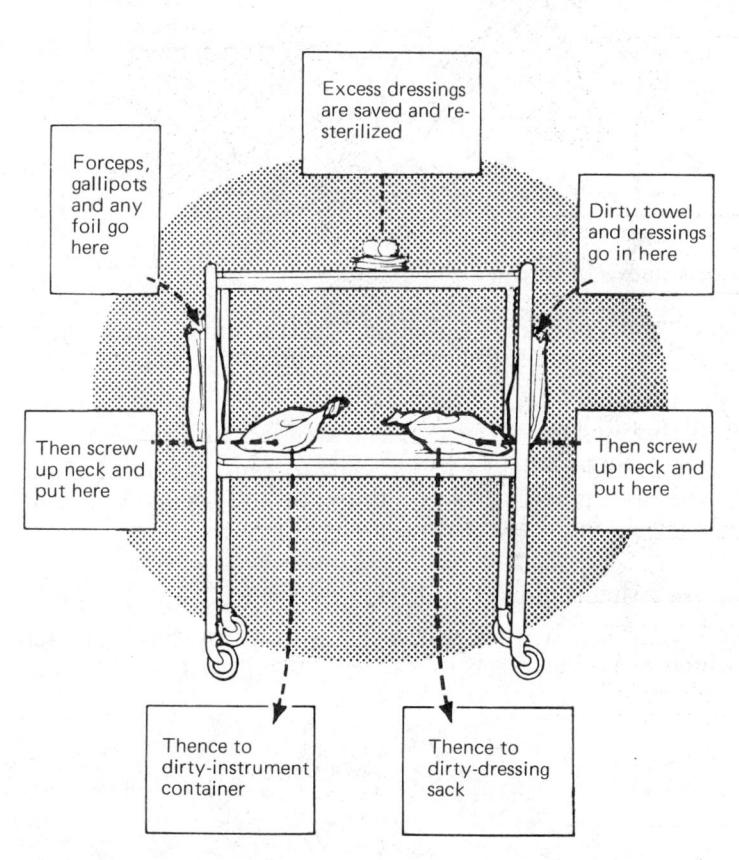

Clearing up

- Excess dressings are saved and re-sterilized
- Forceps, gallipots and any foil go here
- Dirty towel and dressings go in here
- Then screw up neck and put here
- Then screw up neck and put here
- Thence to dirty-instrument container
- Thence to dirty-dressing sack

Fig. 2.d

laying the top shelf, strict aseptic precautions must be observed.

Individual dressing packets containing an inner pack comprising disposable dressing towels, wool swabs, gauze dressings, wool pads and forceps are now in use. The packets are prepared and sterilized in a central sterilizing supply department and supplied to wards and departments as required. Special equipment required for other procedures, such as disposable

148 Practical nursing

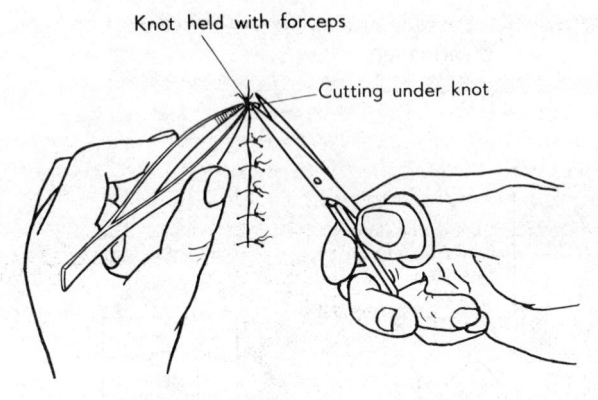

Fig. 15.3 Removal of stitches.

syringes and needles, catheters, instruments, intravenous infusions, etc., are all supplied in presterilized packets.

Removal of stitches

The knot should be held with dressing forceps, the point of the stitch scissors inserted between the knot and the skin and the suture snipped and drawn through (Fig. 15.3).

Removal of Michel clips (Fig. 15.4)

A Michel clip is a strip of soft metal with a tiny tooth at each end which holds the edges of the wound together until healing is complete, usually five to seven days.

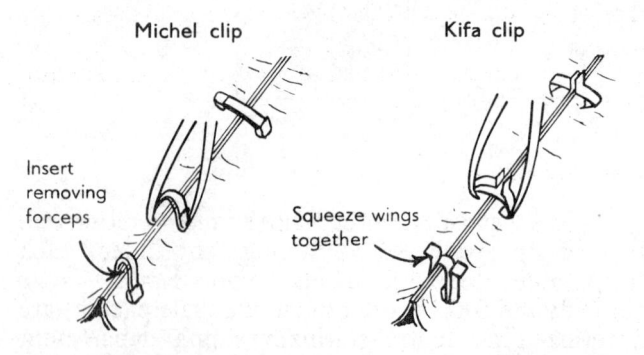

Fig. 15.4 Metal skin clips. (From Nash, D.F.E. *The Principles and Practice of Surgery for Nurses and Allied Professions.* Edward Arnold, London.)

These clips are removed with special clip-removing forceps (see p. 141). The point of the curved blade is carefully inserted underneath the centre of the Michel clip and the forceps gently and firmly closed. The toothed ends rise until the clip is clear of the skin.

The Kifa clip is similar but has two small wings on top which can be pinched together with dressing forceps. This causes the sides of the clip to rise on each side, it can then be removed.

When carried out gently and efficiently, the removal of stitches and clips involves very little pain or discomfort. Nevertheless, most patients are extremely nervous of this procedure and need to be reassured and encouraged to relax.

16
Tissues of the body

Cells and tissues

Every living thing, great or small, is made up of cells, some of which have special functions to perform. They can move about, absorb nourishment and air, throw off waste matter, react to such stimuli as heat, cold, light, etc., and they can reproduce themselves.

When a male and a female cell unite, fertilization takes place and the cells multiply. Each cell divides and subdivides to form other cells, each with its own supply of protoplasm. Cells differ in shape, size and grouping, to form the various tissues that make up the entire body, and throughout life these tissues are constantly repaired and rebuilt with new cells.

The tissues of the body are as follows.
1. Epithelial tissue.
2. Muscular tissue.
3. Nerve tissue.
4. Connective tissue.
5. Bone or osseous tissue.

Epithelial tissue

Epithelial tissue is of two main types, compound and simple epithelium.

Compound epithelium
Compound epithelium consists of several layers of flattened epithelial cells. This covers the outside of the body as skin.

Simple epithelium
The delicate membranes protecting the internal organs of the body are composed of simple epithelium which consists of one layer of cells only and is therefore very thin. These membranes are described as follows.

Tissues of the body

Mucous membrane
Mucous membrane which secretes a thick fluid called *mucus* serving to keep the membrane moist. The respiratory and digestive systems, the urinary bladder and the uterus are all lined with mucous membrane.

Serous membrane
Serous membrane covers most of the abdominal organs, the heart and the lungs. It secretes a serous fluid which acts as a lubricant, allowing the smooth movements of the internal organs.

Synovial membrane
Synovial membrane lines the fibrous capsule surrounding the movable joints. It secretes synovial fluid which acts as a lubricant and allows the joints to move freely.

Ciliated epithelium
In certain areas of the body, some of the membranes have tiny hair-like attachments to each cell called cilia (Fig. 16.1). The cilia have a constant waving motion which sweeps away any irritating substance which may be deposited on the membrane. Ciliated epithelium lines the air passages where dust or mucus may settle. It is also found in the Fallopian tubes of the female reproductive system where it serves to pass the ova into the uterus.

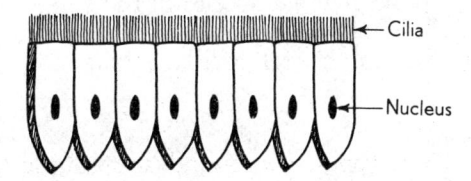

Fig. 16.1 Ciliated epithelium.

Muscular tissue
Muscular tissue is composed of muscle fibres which have the power of contraction (see p. 153).

Nervous tissue
Nervous tissue is made up of nerve cells and nerve fibres which form the brain and spinal cord.

Connective tissue

Connective tissue binds together and supports various parts of the body. The following are examples of connective tissue.

Areolar tissue, found under the skin giving it support.

Adipose tissue, or fat, gives warmth and protection in many parts of the body.

Fibrous tissue which forms ligaments and tendons. (Ligaments support bones, holding them together, and tendons attach muscles to bones).

Elastic tissue stretches and is found in arteries and lungs.

Cartilage, or gristle, is a very tough, pliant tissue. It gives protection in many parts of the body, as in the nose, in the trachea, at the ends of long bones and between the vertebrae. (Discs of cartilage between the vertebrae are called intervertebral discs).

Bone or osseous tissue

Before birth the skeleton is mainly composed of cartilage. After birth special bone cells, together with calcium and phosphorous, are deposited in the cartilage, which gradually becomes hardened.

Growth of bone

Bone cells are laid down in the centre of the shaft of a long bone (the diaphysis) and in the sections of cartilage situated between the ends and the shaft of bone (the epiphyseal cartilages). In this manner the bone grows longer until the child reaches maturity. Injuries to the ends of long bones in children may cause displacement of the epiphyseal cartilage (slipped epiphysis).

17
The muscular system

The muscular system is responsible for all internal and external movements of the body. The muscles are divided into three main types of muscular tissues, each of which differs in its formation according to the work it has to perform. They are:
1. voluntary muscles;
2. involuntary muscles;
3. cardiac muscle.

Voluntary muscles
Voluntary muscles are under the control of the will and enable the body to move freely when required. They are attached to bones by tendons and supplied with nerves which carry impulses from the brain and spinal cord (see p. 158). If these nerves become damaged, the muscles they supply will be paralysed. Voluntary muscles are arranged in pairs, one working in opposition to the other. Those used to bend or *flex* the limbs are known as the *flexors*, while those which straighten the limbs are called *extensors*. (This explains the terms 'flexion' and 'extension'). For example, the biceps muscle on the front of the arm is the flexor, because it pulls the forearm up into the bent position. The triceps muscle on the back of the arm, which straightens it, is the extensor.

Chief voluntary muscles of the body (Fig. 17.1)
    1. The epicranial muscles covering the cranium.
    2. The facial muscles which give expression.
    3. The sterno-mastoid muscles, one on each side of the front of the neck.
    4. The deltoid covering the top of the shoulder.
    5. The trapezius covering the shoulderblades and the back of the neck.
    6. The biceps and triceps of the upper arm.

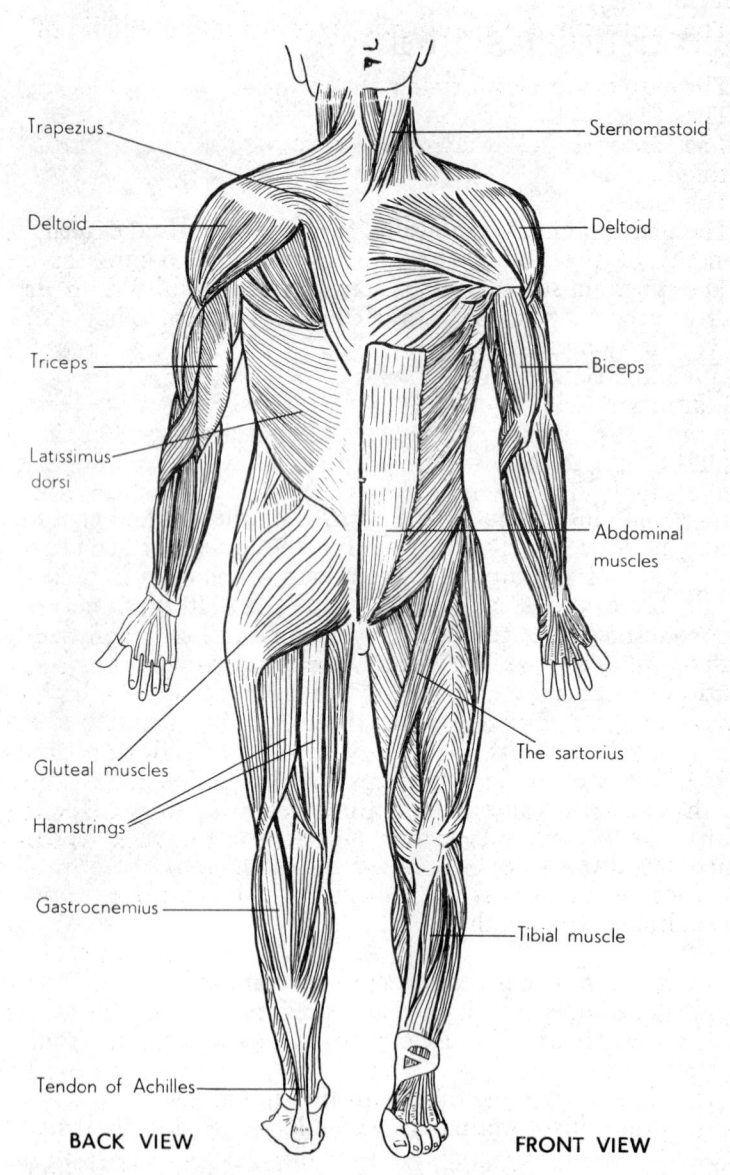

Fig. 17.1 The muscular system. *Left*, back view; *right*, front view.

7. The pectoral muscles over the chest.
8. The intercostal muscles lying between the ribs, which lift them during respiration.
9. The latissimus dorsi, the great muscles at the middle of the back.
10. The gluteal muscles forming the buttocks.
11. The five great muscles forming the abdominal wall.
12. The sartorial and quadriceps muscles covering the front of the thigh.
13. The hamstrings at the back of the thigh.
14. The gastrocnemius at the back of the lower leg (the calf muscle).
15. The tibial muscle over the front of the lower leg.

Involuntary muscles

Involuntary muscles are *not* under the control of the will. They are responsible for the movements of the internal organs of the body such as the stomach, intestines, uterus and other organs. The nerve supply to these involuntary muscles comes from the sympathetic nervous system (see p. 160).

Cardiac muscle

Cardiac muscle is a special type of muscle tissue found only in the wall of the heart and is responsible for the continual beat of the heart throughout life.

Rigor mortis

Immediately after death the muscles remain soft and pliant, but after a time they gradually become stiff and rigid, so that it is impossible to move the limbs without injury to bones and joints. This stiffness is known as rigor mortis and takes place from four to six hours after death.

Disorders affecting muscle tissue

Fibrositis

Fibrositis (muscular rheumatism) is inflammation of muscular tissue causing acute pain, stiffness and limitation of movement. Treatment consists mainly of the application of heat and of massage (physiotherapy). Special liniments may be ordered to be rubbed into the skin over the affected area (inunction).

Lumbago

Lumbago is inflammation of the great muscles of the back in the lumbar region and may be due to injury, exposure, or to an infection in some other part of the body. Treatment is as for fibrositis. In the acute stage complete rest on a hard mattress may be ordered.

Spasm

Spasm is a sudden involuntary contraction of a muscle.

Convulsions are spasms of a general nature, i.e. of the whole body.

Cramp is a painful spasm of a muscle.

Colic is severe pain caused by spasm of involuntary muscle of an internal organ such as the stomach, intestines or ureter.

Tetany

Tetany is a disease characterized by painful contractions and twitching of the muscles. It may affect the face, fingers, toes or the larynx, and may occur as a result of vitamin D deficiency in children or in disorders of the parathyroid glands. After thyroidectomy, the patient is closely observed for signs of twitching of the muscles of the face. This may denote that, as a result of surgical interference, the function of the parathyroid glands has been impaired (see p. 117). The muscular contractions may last from a few minutes to several hours.

18
The brain and the nervous system

The brain is situated in the cranium and consists of nerve cells (the grey matter) and nerve fibres (the white matter).

The main parts of the brain (Fig 18.1) are:
the cerebrum or larger brain;
the cerebellum or lesser brain;
the pons varolii;
the medulla oblongata.

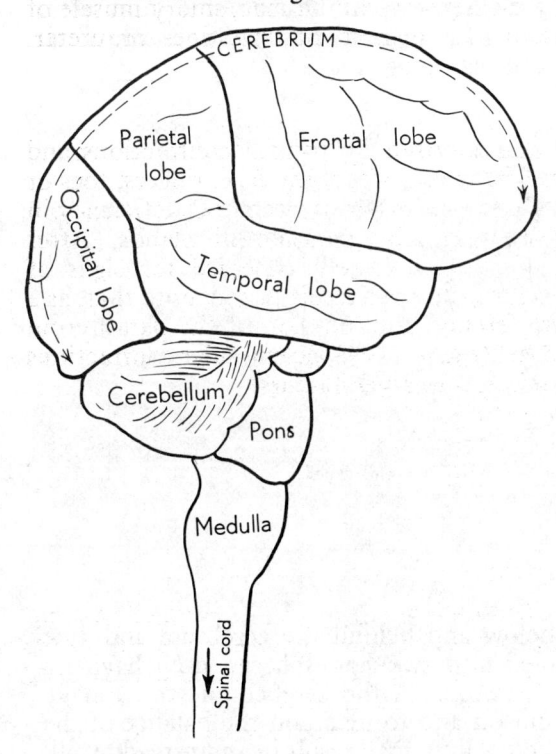

Fig. 18.1 The brain.

The cerebrum

The cerebrum is situated largely in the top and front of the cranium. Its surface is drawn up into folds, or convolutions, and it is divided by a deep grove, running from front to back, into the right and left cerebral hemishperes. In each hemisphere is a cavity, known as a ventricle, containing cerebrospinal fluid. The cerebrum is divided into lobes which contain the following various nerve centres, making it one of the most active parts of the brain.

1. The motor centres controlling the voluntary muscles of the body. Each hemisphere controls the muscles on the opposite side of the body, e.g. injury to the right side of the brain causes paralysis of the left side of the body and vice versa.

2. The sensory centres carrying sensations of touch, pain, heat and cold to the skin and to a lesser extent to muscles and bones.

3. The centres of special sense, sight, hearing, smell and taste.

4. The centres of higher mental powers, consciousness, memory, intelligence and reasoning (Fig. 18.2).

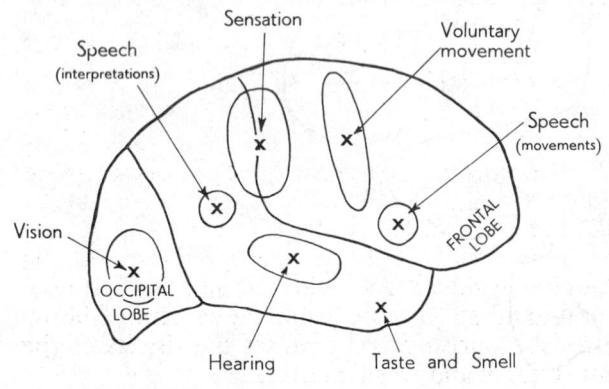

Fig. 18.2 The cerebrum.

The cerebellum

The cerebellum lies below and behind the cerebrum and, like the cerebrum, is divided into two hemispheres, each having a pleated surface. The functions of the cerebellum are to make the muscles work in unison and to maintain the balance of the body. Disease of the cerebellum may result in an unsteady walk and difficulty in holding things securely.

The pons varolii

The pons varolii forms a bridge of nerve fibres connecting the two sides of the cerebellum.

The medulla oblongata

The medulla oblongata is continuous with the pons varolii, forming a link between the brain and spinal cord. It lies just inside the foramen magnum, the opening in the occiput at the base of the skull. In the medulla are the vital reflex centres of life, the cardiac and respiratory centres and those controlling the actions of swallowing, vomiting and coughing.

The meninges

This is the name given to the three protective membranes covering the brain and spinal cord.
 1. *The dura mater,* the tough outer coat, lying between the arachnoid membrane and the hard, bony surface of the inside of the skull. This coat covers the entire brain, and is folded between the cerebrum and the cerebellum to give protection and support.
 2. *The arachnoid membrane,* the serous, middle covering of the brain which serves to hold cerebrospinal fluid.
 3. *The pia mater,* a thin delicate membrane made up almost entirely of tiny blood vessels by which the brain receives its blood supply. This membrane covers the surface of the brain very closely, dipping down into all the crevices and convolutions.
 Cerebrospinal fluid is a clear, watery fluid stored in the ventricles of the brain and held in the space between the pia mater and the arachnoid membrane, where it acts as a cushion, protecting the brain and spinal cord from the effects of blows or concussion. It also nourishes and cleanses the tissues of the brain, carrying away toxic and waste matter.

The cranial nerves

There are twelve pairs of nerves leaving the brain. Some are motor, carrying messages from the brain to the muscles, and some are mixed nerves carrying messages to and from the brain. The cranial nerves include the nerves of smell, sight, hearing and taste and those responsible for movements of the face, tongue and neck. One of the most important of these is the *vagus* nerve which controls the activity of the pharynx, larynx, trachea, bronchi, lungs, heart, oesophagus, stomach and the upper part of the intestines. After leaving the brain it passes through the thorax, through the diaphragm and into the abdominal cavity.

The spinal cord

This is a cylinder of nerve tissue, about the thickness of the little finger and some 40-45 cm (16-18 in) long. It passes out from the brain through the opening at the base of the occiput, known as the foramen magnum, and is contained in the bony canal formed by the neural arches of the vertebrae (see p. 179). It is covered by the meninges and the cerebrospinal fluid in the same manner as the brain. From the spinal cord, thirty-one pairs of spinal nerves are given off, which carry impulses to and from the brain to control the muscles of the limbs and trunk. These are divided into the following groups:

    8 pairs of cervical nerves;
   12 pairs of dorsal nerves;
    5 pairs of lumbar nerves;
    5 pairs of sacral nerves;
    1 pair of coccygeal nerves.

The autonomic or sympathetic nervous system

This system of nerves acts automatically and is divided into two parts.
    (a) The parasympathetic nervous system.
    (b) The sympathetic nervous system.

The parasympathetic nervous system

The parasympathetic nervous system gives off branches to the internal organs of the body, chiefly by the vagus nerve which passes through the thorax, pierces the diaphragm and descends into the abdominal cavity. Other nerves of this system control the action of the eyes and the salivary glands. The parasympathetic nervous system is in control during the normal working of the body.

The sympathetic nervous system

The sympathetic nervous system also gives off branches to the internal organs, but is stimulated into action by strong emotion, such as fear, anger, or excitement, giving rise to the desire to run away from danger or to stand and fight. Disturbance of the normal functioning of the internal organs, causing symptoms of indigestion, vomiting, respiratory distress, etc., may also arise as a result of over-activity of the sympathetic nervous system. Each organ in the body receives a nerve supply from both systems, the sympathetic nervous system stimulating and the parasympathetic nervous system checking the action of the organs.

Common diseases of the brain

Apoplexy is the term used to describe the sudden unconsciousness often accompanied by paralysis, connected with diseases of the brain. Such an attack is commonly known as a stroke and mostly occurs in middle-aged or elderly people. General signs and symptoms are cyanosis, stridor (noisy respirations), incontinence, paralysis, loss of speech and unconsciousness.

Cerebral haemorrhage is the escape of blood from a damaged blood vessel in the brain, causing increasing pressure on the brain.

Cerebral thrombosis is a condition in which a clot of blood forms in a diseased artery in the brain.

Cerebral embolism occurs as the result of a clot breaking away from a diseased blood vessel in some other part of the body, or from a diseased area in the left side of the heart. The detached clot is carried round in the bloodstream until it reaches the brain, where it becomes lodged in an artery. An embolus may also consist of an air bubble or of fragments of fatty tissue.

Cerebral tumours produce pressure on the brain. Symptoms vary according to the site of the tumour and may include headache, vomiting, changes in behaviour or visual disturbances, followed by the general signs and symptoms described above.

Paralysis

Types of paralysis
Monoplegia is paralysis on one limb or one set of muscles.

Hemiplegia (Fig. 18.3) is paralysis of one side of the body.

Paraplegia (Fig. 18.4) is paralysis of the lower part of the trunk and the legs, usually as a result of disease or injury of the spinal cord.

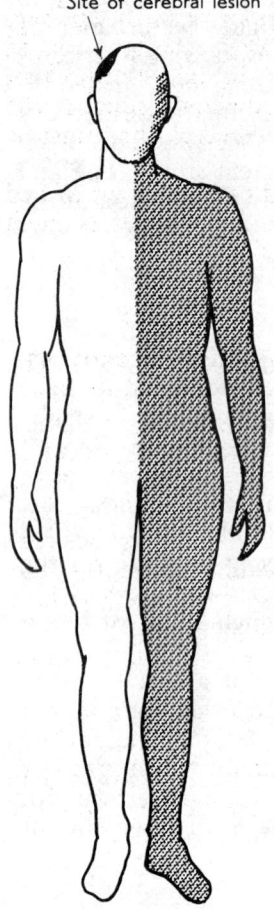

Fig. 18.3 Hemiplegia.

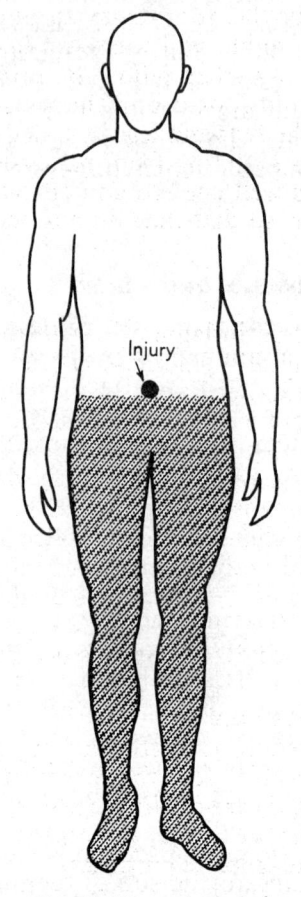

Fig. 18.4 Paraplegia below point of spinal injury.

Nursing care
Nursing care at the onset of diseases of the brain will include rest in bed, frequent change of position to avoid risk of hypo static pneumonia (see p. 54), warmth without overheating, regular mouth hygiene, daily bed-baths, especially where the patient is incontinent, strict attention to pressure areas and, for the conscious patient, a light nourishing diet. Unconscious patients will be artificially fed (see p. 109). Careful watch must

also be kept on the bladder for either incontinence or retention of urine. Paralysed legs should be well supported with sandbags to prevent the foot from turning outwards. A pillow placed under the ankle will raise the heel from the bed and prevent bed-sores. Another pillow or a foot board should support the feet to avoid foot drop. The weight of the bed-clothes must be kept off the feet and legs by a bed cradle.

Patients suffering from paralysis should be helped out of bed as soon as well enough and encouraged to move about as much as possible, so that they do not become bedridden.

Meningitis

Meningitis is inflammation of the meninges (se p. 159). The patient rapidly becomes very ill with severe headaches, rigor, hyperpyrexia, stiffness of the muscles of the neck and limbs, mental confusion, and irritability. Convulsions may occur in children.

Nursing care   The patient should be nursed in a darkened room and absolute quiet maintained. The nursing position should be changed and pressure areas treated frequently. The diet should be light and nourishing with plenty of fluids. Where swallowing is difficult, naso-gastric feeding may become necessary (see p. 109). Lumbar puncture is usually carried out to identify the causative organism.

Lumbar puncture

This procedure is performed by a doctor, but the nurse may be responsible for the preparation of the trolley and the position and care of the patient.

   Reasons for lumbar puncture
   1. For diagnostic purposes.
   2. To relieve the pressure of fluid on the brain.
   3. To estimate the pressure of the cerebrospinal fluid.
   4. To introduce anaesthetics or other drugs into the body.

This procedure is carried out with the strictest aseptic precautions. The patient must be reassured and the procedure explained as far as possible. The left lateral position is adopted, with the knees drawn well up towards the chin and the head bent towards the chest, so that the spine is fully flexed and the lumbar vertebrae separated. The patient must be supported in this position throughout the procedure. A local anaesthetic is injected into the lumbar region before the lumbar puncture is carried out.

Requirements

Trolley with:
special lumbar puncture pack, or
dressing pack;
selection of disposable lumbar puncture needles;
manometer (Fig. 18.5);
specimen bottles as required (usually two or three);
skin-cleansing lotion;
local anaesthetic;
2-ml syringe;
hypodermic needles;
sterile gloves;

Manometer

Lumbar puncture needle with tap

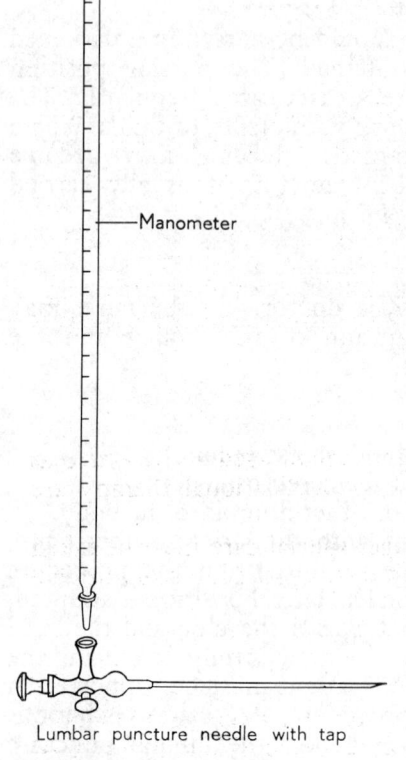

Fig. 18.5 Manometer.

masks (as necessary);
Nobecutane spray (for sealing punctures)
elastoplast dressing;
any drugs for injections and prescription sheet.
In addition:
good lighting;
stool for doctor;
receptacle for soiled articles;
blanket for patient.

After lumbar puncture the patient should be made comfortable and the foot of the bed raised on blocks. If fluid has been withdrawn, this position prevents the headache which might result from loss of cerebrospinal fluid from the ventricle of the brain. Where drugs have been injected into the spinal cord, this position allows the upward flow to the brain.

Common diseases affecting the nervous system

Multiple sclerosis

Multiple sclerosis is a disease of unknown origin attacking and destroying the myelin sheath which protects the nerve fibres of the central nervous system. This causes muscular spasms and rigidity of the limbs, difficulty in walking and tremor of the hands. At a later stage, there is blurring of speech and nystagmus (involuntary rapid movement of the eye). The disease is incurable, but there may be long periods of remission when some or all of the symptoms subside and the patient is comparatively well.

Nursing care
The patient must be reassured and encouraged to be active as long as possible. Physiotherapy and occupational therapy are invaluable in attaining this end.

During the later bed-ridden stage, special care must be taken in the prevention of bed-sores and in the provision of a nourishing, easily digested diet.

Epilepsy

Epilepsy is a condition which usually begins during childhood, but attacks may occur at any age. There are two types of epilepsy, minor and major.

(a) Minor epilepsy (petit mal) is more common than the major type. The patient becomes momentarily unconscious but recovers almost immediately and is often unaware that anything unusual has happened.

(b) Major epilepsy occurs in four stages.

1. *The warning stage* in which the patient may be aware of peculiar sensations, nausea, noises, etc., commonly known as the 'aura'.

2. *The rigid stage* in which the patient becomes rigid and unconscious and falls. The teeth are clenched and the tongue may be bitten. The face is cyanosed. During this stage breathing may stop for a few seconds.

3. *The convulsive stage* in which the muscles twitch, the tongue may be bitten and there is frothing at the mouth. Urine or faeces may be involuntarily passed at this stage.

4. *The comatosed stage* in which the patient becomes deeply unconscious then rapidly passes into deep sleep.

The post-epileptic state

On recovering from the fit, the patient may appear quite normal and carry on with his usual occupation, but will not remember what he has been doing. It is therefore important, in view of this loss of memory, that the epileptic patient is watched carefully for some time following a major fit.

Treatment

All tight clothing should be loosened and the head turned to one side. The patient must be prevented from knocking himself, and the jaws should be slightly opened by placing a spatula, or in emergency, the handle of a spoon, between the back teeth to prevent the tongue from being bitten. Force should not be used in restraining the patient as this might lead to injury. When the attack has passed, the patient should be kept quiet and, where possible, left to rest.

Herpes zoster (shingles)

Herbes zoster (shingles) is a disease caused by a virus infection of a nerve, usually in the intercostal area, although it may also occur on the face. It is marked by severe pain, followed by the appearance of a rash along the course of a nerve. Later, vesicles form over the area and eventually become crusted.

Treatment The patient is confined to bed and kept as quiet as possible. Freedom from anxiety is important. The affected areas are kept dry and lightly powdered and sedatives given as ordered. The pain may last for several weeks, particularly in elderly patients, making them feel miserable and depressed. Constant reassurance is needed to overcome this condition.

Sciatica

Sciatica is inflammation of the sciatic nerve and may be caused by cold and dampness or by a prolapsed intervertebral disc (see p. 192).

Treatment Rest and warmth are important in the relief of the acute pain of sciatica. Splints and sandbags should be used to prevent undue movement of the affected limb. Where the pain is caused by a prolapsed intervertebral disc, the patient is nursed flat on the back and great care must be taken, when lifting or turning the patient, to avoid aggravating the pain.

19
The eye

The eye lies in the socket known as the orbit and rests on a cushion of fat which protects it from injury by blows or pressure. The eyelids and eyebrows also serve to protect the eyeball.

The eyelids

The eyelids are lined with a transparent membrane called the *conjunctiva* which is folded back to cover the white of the eye. The conjunctiva contains nerves and many tiny blood vessels which dilate if the eye is irritated or injured, causing it to become bloodshot.

The lacrimal glands

The lacrimal gland lies in the upper and outer corner of the orbit. It continually secretes a clear, watery fluid which passes over the surface of the eye, keeping it clear and moist. The fluid escapes into the nose through the *lacrimal duct,* at the inner corner of the orbit. Over-secretion by the lacrimal gland causes the fluid to overflow on to the cheeks as tears (Fig. 19.1).

The eyeball

The eyeball has three coats, the *sclerotic,* the *choroid* and the *retina.*
　1. *The sclerotic and the cornea.* The sclerotic is the thickest coat and forms the outer, white part of the eye. It is composed of a strong, fibrous membrane, except in front where it bulges to form the circular transparent *cornea* which protects the lens and through which light rays enter.
　2. *The choroid and the iris.* The choroid is a dark coat containing black colouring matter which darkens the chamber of the eye and prevents the reflection of light inside the eye. In front, the choroid becomes the *iris,* the circular, coloured

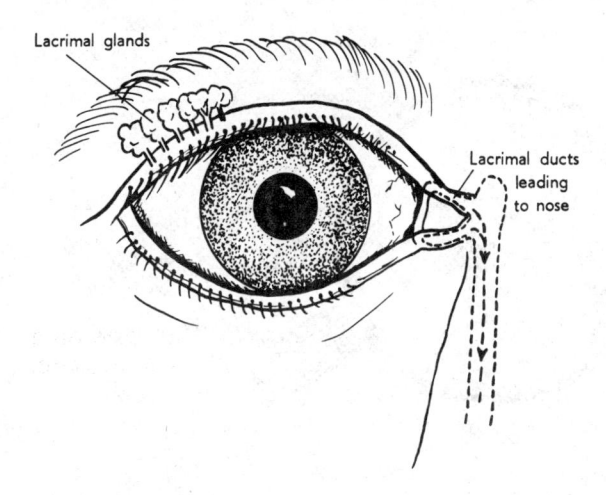

Fig. 19.1 The lacrimal glands and ducts.

portion seen through the transparent cornea. In the centre of the iris is the small hole known as the *pupil* through which light rays pass into the eye. The iris is provided with sets of tiny muscles which dilate and contract the pupil, thus controlling the amount of light entering the eye and falling on the lens. In bright light the pupil contracts to shut out some of the rays and when the light is dim or the vision is focused on distant objects the pupil dilates to allow more light to enter.

3. *The retina* is the innermost coat of the eyeball formed by an expansion of the optic nerve which enters at the back and a little to the nasal side of the eye. The retina is a delicate membrane, made up of nerve fibres and specialized nerve endings, which form impressions of light and colour *from the outside world*. These impressions are carried by the optic nerve to the brain where they are transformed into vision as we know it.

The lens

The lens lies close behind the iris and is enclosed in a capsule held firmly in place by the *suspensory ligaments*. The lens serves to focus rays of light on to the retina, but the amount of light passing through the lens depends on the size of the pupil.

Between the cornea and the lens is a cavity known as the anterior chamber which is filled with a clear, watery fluid called *aqueous humour*. Behind the lens is a larger cavity filled with a

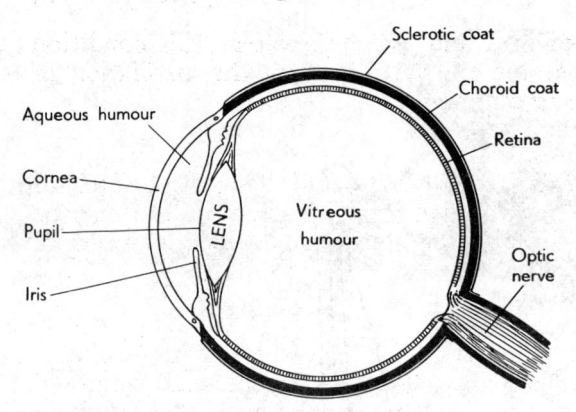

Fig. 19.2 The eye.

jelly-like substance called *vitreous humour*. These fluids give the eyeball its shape and help to keep it firm (Fig. 19.2).

Some disorders of the eye

Blepharitis
Blepharitis is inflammation of the edges of the eyelids, causing them to become sore, red and sticky. The lids may become adherent.

Treatment
The eyelids are bathed with sodium chloride eye lotion and the edges smeared with simple eye ointment to remove crusts.

Cataract
Cataract is an opaque film which forms within the lens, causing loss of vision. Surgical treatment is often carried out and the diseased lens removed.

Conjunctivitis
Conjunctivitis is inflammation of the conjunctiva caused by grit or other foreign bodies, by irritation, by viruses, by bacteria or by exposure of the eyes to strong sunlight. The conjunctiva

becomes red and painful and the eyes water. This condition may be acute or chronic and is treated by the instillation of antibiotic eye drops or ointment.

Purulent conjunctivitis
Purulent conjunctivitis is a severe and dangerous form of conjunctivitis in which the sight may be affected, and may be caused by infection of the eyes of the newborn by venereal disease of the mother.

Pink eye
Pink eye is a highly infective form of conjunctivitis, due to a specific type of bacteria. It may appear in epidemic form and can be spread by the use of communal towels and handkerchiefs. Should an outbreak of pink eye occur amongst schoolchildren, the schools may be closed by order of the Medical Officer of Health (see p. 129).

A stye

A stye is caused by the infection of a follicle of an eyelash. Pus forms and appears as a septic spot on the edge of the eyelid, giving rise to a hard, round and painful swelling with oedema of the eyelid. Antibiotics may be ordered.

Care of artificial eyes

These are expensive and should be treated with great care. The artificial eye should be removed from the socket each day and washed and rinsed thoroughly before being replaced. The socket should be bathed with warm sterile saline. Where the patient is to go to the theatre, the artificial eye should be removed, put into distilled water and left in a safe place until the patient has fully recovered from the anaesthetic.

Nursing treatment of the eye

Hot spooning in which the eyelids are steamed first.

Requirements
Wooden spoon, the bowl of the spoon is padded with cotton wool secured with cotton bandage.
    Jug of very hot water.
    Wool swabs in a bowl, receiver for soiled swabs.
    Small towel for the face.

Method The bowl or jug with the padded spoon is placed on a tray on the bed-table in front of the patient. The patient is instructed to hold the spoon in front of, but not touching, the closed eye, so that the steam circulates over the eyelids. As the water cools it should be replaced with hot water and the process continued for ten to fifteen minutes. The eyelids are then swabbed from the inner corner to the outer corner, using each swab once only, and left as dry as possible.

Irrigation of the eye

Requirements
Undine standing in a small bowl, bowl of wool swabs.
Jug of normal saline, temperature 37°C (99°F).
Lotion thermometer.
Receiver in which to collect the lotion, receiver for soiled swabs.
Waterproof cape and towel.

Method
The patient's head is turned with the affected eye on the lower side and the waterproof and towel placed under the side of the face. The receiver for collecting the lotion is held against the cheek with a pad of wool to protect the skin. Usually this can be done by the patient, but where this is not possible a second nurse will be required to assist. The lotion should be poured first over the upper part of the cheek and then on to the eye, allowing the fluid to flow away from the inner corner of the orbit. The patient should be instructed to keep both eyes open and to look upwards while the lower lid is drawn gently downwards, to that the lotion comes into contact with all parts of the conjunctiva. When irrigation is complete, the eyelids should be cleansed and dried, using each swab once only, and left clean and free of secretions.

Instillation of eye drops

These are now prepared in single-dose units and are taken to the bedside on a tray with wool swabs and the prescription sheet.
Care must be taken that the correct type, strength and number of drops are inserted.

Method
The nurse should stand behind the patient where possible and the patient should be instructed to look upwards whilst the lower lid is drawn downwards and the drops placed gently inside the lower lid. Drops should not be allowed to fall directly on to the cornea or the patient may close the eyes tightly making the procedure more difficult.

20
The ear

The ear is divided into three parts, the outer ear consisting of the *pinna* and the *external auditory canal*, the middle ear and inner ear (Fig. 20.1a).

The outer ear

The pinna is situated outside the head and is specially adapted to collect sound waves which then pass along the external auditory canal. The walls of this canal are provided with tiny hairs near the opening which prevent the entrance of insects into the ear, and with glands which secrete wax which protects the ear by trapping dust, dirt or insects. The inner end of the auditory canal is closed by a membrane called the *tympanum* or *ear drum*, which separates the outer ear from the middle ear.

The middle ear

The middle ear (Fig 20.1c) is a tiny cavity in the temporal bone, separated from the inner ear by a thin wall of bone in which are two small openings, each covered with membrane. Because of their shape, these openings are known as the round and oval windows.

The middle ear contains a chain of three minute bones called collectively the *ossicles*, although each has its own name. They are as follows.

1. The mallet, because it resembles a hammer. The handle of the mallet is attached to the inner side of the ear drum.

2. The incus, or anvil, on which the head of the mallet rests.

3. The stapes, or stirrup bone, so called because it resembles a horse's stirrup.

The incus is attached to the stapes and the foot piece of the stapes is attached to the membrane covering the oval window (see above).

From the floor of the middle ear, the Eustachian tube opens

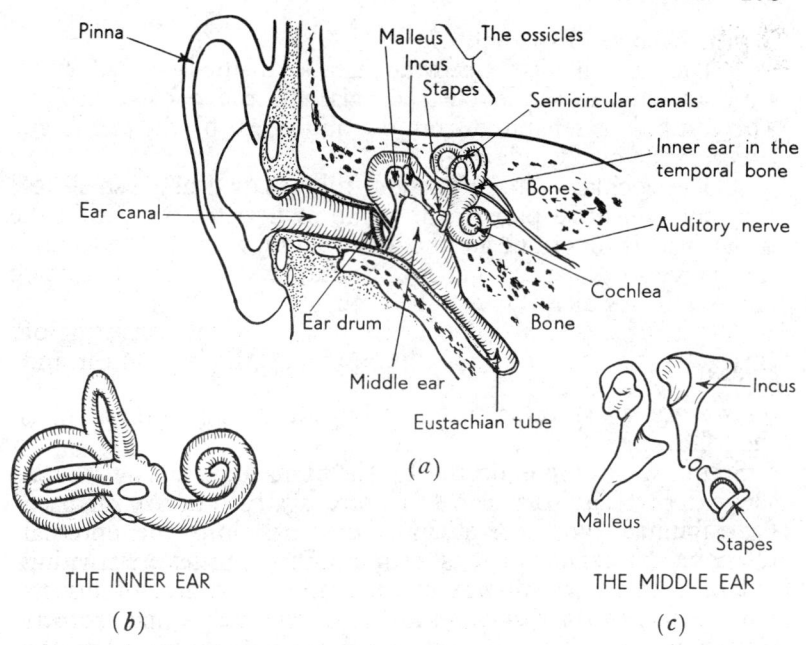

Fig. 20.1 The ear; (a) complete, (b) inner, (c) middle.

to communicate with the pharynx (see p. 96). Through the Eustachian tube the pressure of air in the middle ear is adjusted by the action of swallowing. From the side of the middle ear a second opening is connected with the antrum of the mastoid process of the temporal bone.

The inner ear

The inner ear (Fig. 20.1b) is situated deep inside the temporal bone where it is well protected. It is separated from the middle ear by the thin wall of bone in which the round and oval windows are placed. The inner ear consists of a series of tiny, bony cavities forming the *bony labyrinth*, which is made up of three parts.

1. The semicircular canals, which are concerned with the sense of position and balance of the body. These bony canals are lined with membrane and contain fluid. The fluid moves with every movement of the head to stimulate the nerve endings of balance which communicate with the brain. (It will be remembered that the cerebellum is also concerned with maintain-

ing the balance of the body.) (See p. 158).

2. The vestibule is the central chamber of the bony labyrinth, from which the semicircular canals and the cochlea project. The vestibule is separated from the middle ear by the membrane covering the oval window.

3. The cochlea is a bony, spiral tube shaped like a shell. It is the most sensitive part of the organ of hearing, for within the spiral of this tiny bone are the nerve endings which join to form the nerve of hearing, called the auditory nerve. This nerve communicates directly with the brain.

Hearing

Sound waves are transmitted through the ears to the brain in the following manner.

Sound waves are collected by the pinna and, passing through the external auditory canal, vibrate against the ear drum or tympanum. From the tympanum they pass into the middle ear to shake the ossicles. The vibrations of the ossicles are transmitted through the membrane covering the oval window, into the inner ear, and on through the bony labyrinth to the cochlea. Here they are picked up by the auditory nerve in the cochlea and passed to the centre of hearing in the temporal lobe of the brain, where they are translated into sounds which can be recognized and understood.

21
The skeleton

Bone structure

There are two distinct kinds of bone tissue which can be clearly seen in the bones of the skeleton. The outer portion of a bone is composed of an extremely hard, ivory-like substance called *compact bone tissue*. Underneath this compact layer is a spongy, porous bone called *cancellous tissue* which serves to lessen the weight of bone.

Varities of bone

Because the bones of the skeleton vary in shape they are classified for easy recognition as follows.
 1. Long bones, as the arms and legs.
 2. Short bones, as of the wrist and ankle.
 3. Flat bones as of the top of the skull.
 4. Irregular bones as of the spine.

Long bones consist of a central, hollow shaft, with a rounded portion at each end. The walls of the shaft are composed of compact bone. The ends of the long bones have an outer shell of compact bone filled with cancellous, or spongy, bone. The hollow shaft contains yellow bone marrow. In the spaces of the cancellous tissue at the ends of long bones, red marrow is found. (Blood cells are manufactured in bone marrow.)

Short and irregular bones have no shaft and consist of a thin outer layer of compact bone tissue filled in with cancellous tissue.

Flat bones are made up of a layer of cancellous bone between two layers of compact bone.

Periosteum

This is a tough, fibrous membrane closely covering the surface of all bones except where they form part of a joint, as at the ends of the long bones. Blood is carried into the bone by small

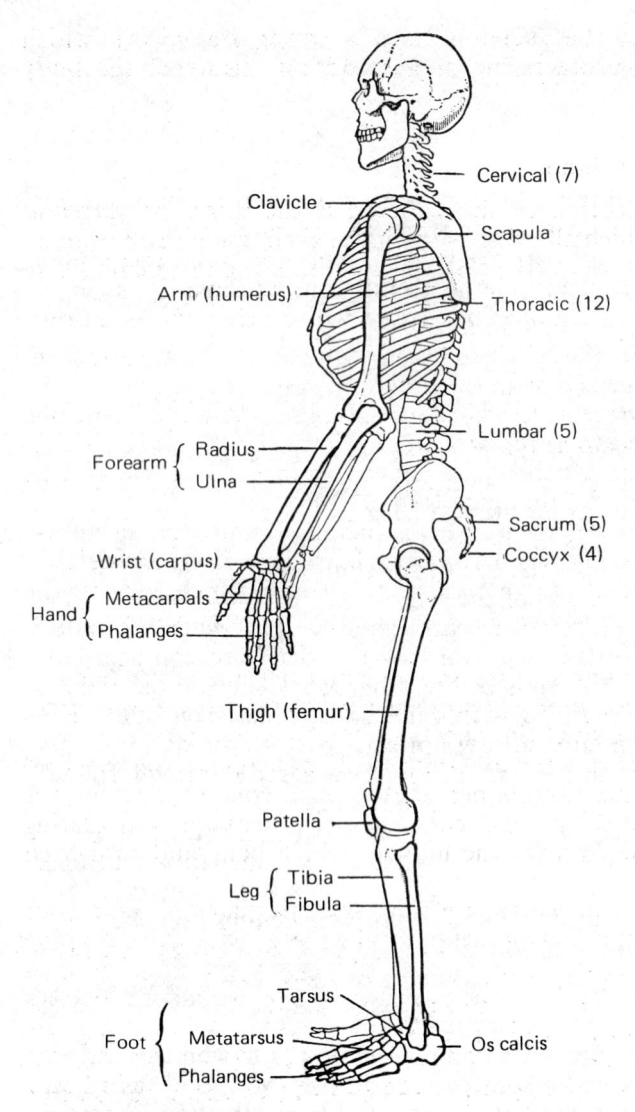

Fig. 21.1 The skeleton.

blood vessels from the periosteum. If the periosteum is destroyed, the circulation of blood is cut off from the underlying part of the bone which then becomes diseased.

The skeleton

The bones of the skeleton form a strong framework which supports and protects the organs and soft tissue of the body (Fig. 21.1).

The vertebral column

The central portion of the skeleton is the spinal or *vertebral column*, to which all other parts of the skeleton are connected.

This consists of thirty-three small bones called vertebrae. These are divided into groups as follows.

7 cervical vertebrae in the neck.

12 dorsal or thoracic vertebrae to which the ribs are attached.

5 lumbar vertebrae in the loin.

5 sacral vertebrae, which in the adult are united into one bony plate known as *the sacrum.*

4 coccygeal vertebrae also joined together to form the *coccyx* at the lower end of the spine (Fig. 21.2).

Each of the vertebrae is constructed on the same principle, although differing slightly in detail. A vertebra consists of a bony mass called the *body* in front, an *arch,* which encloses the spinal cavity or *neural canal* (Fig. 21.3). (The spinal cord runs through this canal.)

The transverse processes arise one on each side of the body.

The spinous process projects backwards from the arch, opposite the body of the vertebrae.

These processes serve as places of attachment for the ligaments which hold the bones of the spinal column together, for the tendons of the muscles connected to other bones articulating with the spine, and for the muscles which bend and straighten the body.

The articular processes are tiny, smooth plates of bone, four on each vertebra. These articulate, or join, with the vertebrae immediately above and below, except in the first cervical vertebra (the atlas) where the two upper articular processes correspond with those on the base of the skull.

Invertebral discs are thick pads of cartilage between each of the vertebrae in the three upper groups, i.e. the cervical, the thoracic and the lumbar vertebrae. These discs allow freedom

180 *Practical nursing*

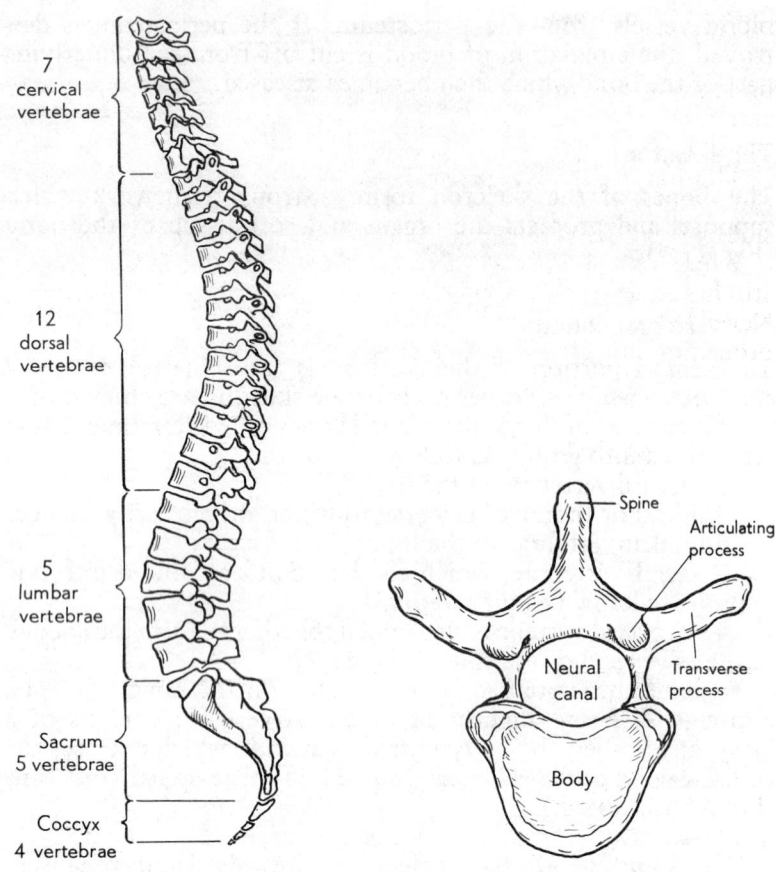

Fig. 21.2 Vertebral column.

Fig. 21.3 A typical vertebra.

of movement and act as buffers to prevent shock or jarring of the spine.

Special vertebrae
The two top vertebrae are a little different in formation from the others. The first vertebra on which the skull rests is called *the atlas* (Fig. 21.4). It is ring shaped and has no body. On its upper surface are two smooth plates of bone on which the skull rests. The second cervical vertebra, the *axis* (Fig. 21.5), has a tooth-like peg projecting upwards, called the *odontoid process.* This peg acts as the axis round which the atlas moves, allowing the head to be turned from side to side.

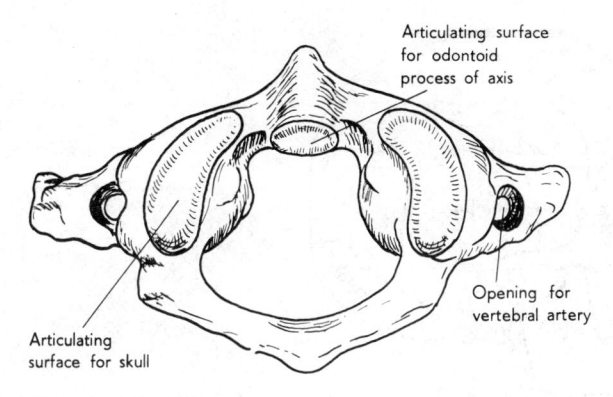

Fig. 21.4 The atlas.

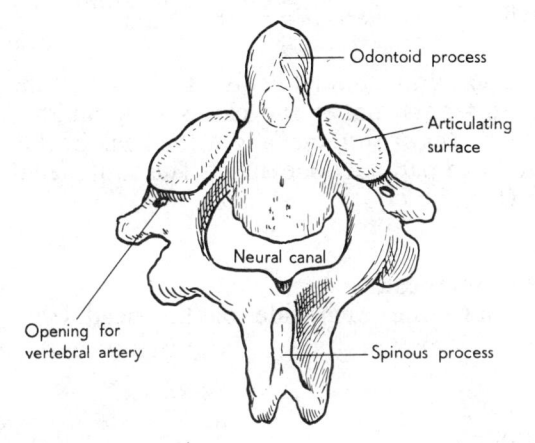

Fig. 21.5 The axis.

The skull

The skull is balanced on top of the vertebral column, resting on the atlas as described above, It consists of the cranium and the bones of the face. The cranium is the large, hollow, bony case which encloses the brain. The bones of the face form the front and lower part of the skull (Fig. 21.6).

The cranium is made up eight flat bones firmly joined together by saw-like edges, calles sutures. In the adult the bones of the cranium cannot be moved. In infancy these bones are not firmly joined but are connected by a membrane which allows for expansion as the child grows. The membranous spaces are

182 *Practical nursing*

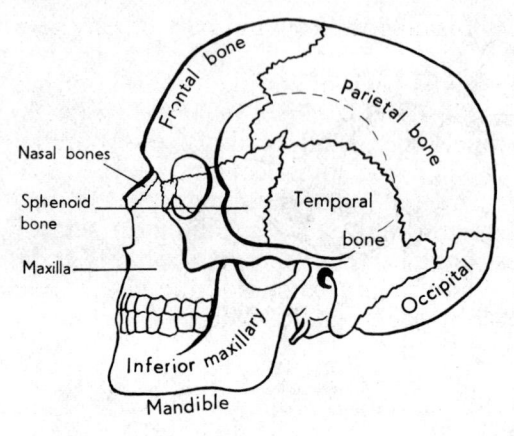

Fig. 21.6 Bones of the skull.

called fontanelles. The *anterior fontanelle* is at the junction between the parietal and frontal bones and closes at about the age of 18 months. The *posterior fontanelle* is at the back of the skull where the occipital and parietal bones meet. This fontanelle closes soon after birth (Fig. 21.7).

Bones of the cranium
  1. *The frontal bone* or forehead.
  2. *Two temporal bones,* one each side of the head (the temples).

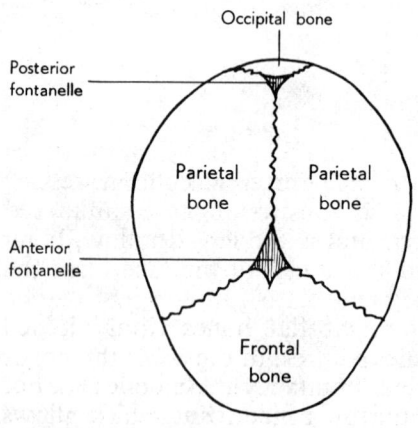

Fig. 21.7 The cranium.

3. *Two parietal bones* forming the top and part of the sides of the skull.

4. *The occipital bone* at the back of the skull. This bone has an opening in its base called the *foramen magnum* (meaning 'large hole') through which the spinal cord passes from the brain into the neural canal of the spinal column (see p. 160).

5. *The ethmoid bone,* situated inside the skull and separating the cavity of the nose from the brain. It has many small openings through which branches of the nerve of smell pass into the brain.

6. *The sphenoid bone* is also situated inside the base of the skull and resembles a bat with outstretched wings.

Bones of the face
There are fourteen bones in the face, as follows.

1. Two *malar,* or *cheek, bones.*

2. Two *lacrimal bones,* one at each inner corner of the eye sockets. These contain the lacrimal ducts (tear ducts) which carry tears away from the eyes into the nasal cavities.

3. The *vomer* in the nose, separating the nostrils.

4. Two *nasal bones* forming the upper part of the bridge of the nose.

5. Two *turbinated bones,* one in each nostril.

6. Two *palate bones* forming the hard palate in the mouth.

7. Two *superior maxillary bones* joined in the centre to form the upper jaw.

8. One *inferior maxillary bone,* the lower jaw, sometimes called the mandible.

The hyoid bone is a small, U-shaped bone situated above the trachea. It supports the tongue which is attached to it by ligaments and muscles.

Bones of the thorax

The thorax, or chest, is a cavity containing the heart, the lungs, the bronchial tubes, the trachea, the oesophagus (the food pipe), the thoracic duct (the largest lymphatic duct in the body) and the great nerves and blood vessels. All these vital organs are protected by a bony cage formed by the following structures.

1. The *sternum* in front of the chest. This is a soft dagger-shaped bone to which some of the ribs are connected. The lower end of the sternum is composed of cartilage.

2. The *ribs,* of which there are twelve pairs, are all attached to the dorsal vertebrae at the back of the thorax. The upper seven pairs are known as the 'true ribs', because they are

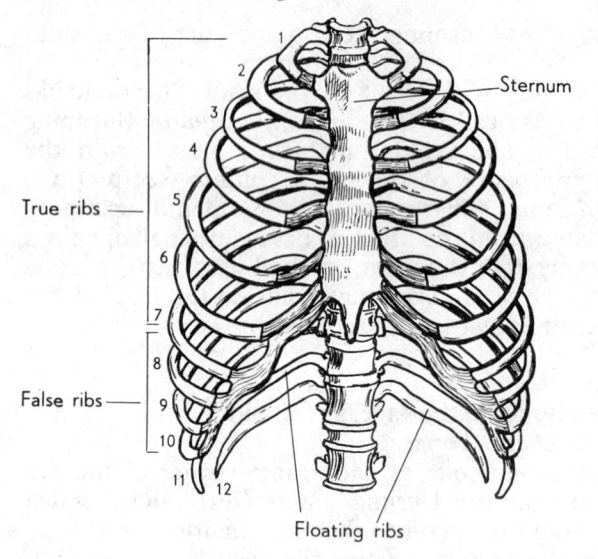

Fig. 21.8 Rib cage with sternum.

connected by *separate* pieces of cartilage to the sternum in front. The lower five pairs are called 'false ribs'. Of these, the three upper pairs are connected to the sternum by *one* piece of cartilage. The last two pairs are not attached in front and are termed 'floating' ribs (Fig. 21.8).

The shoulder girdle and upper limbs

The bones of the shoulder girdle (Fig 21.9) are the *clavicle* (the collar bone) and the *scapula* (the shoulder-blade).

The *clavicle* articulates with the top of the sternum at one end and at the other it forms a joint with the shoulder-blade.

The *scapula*, or shoulder-blade, is a triangular bone lying outside the rib cage. At the upper and outer end is a hollow called the *glenoid cavity*, into which the head of the *humerus* fits to form the shoulder joint.

Bones of the arm
The *humerus* is the bone of the upper arm, extending from the shoulder to the elbow. It is a long bone with rounded ends. The upper head fits into the scapula, as described above, to form a ball and socket joint at the shoulder. The lower end of the humerus articulates with the bones of the forearm.

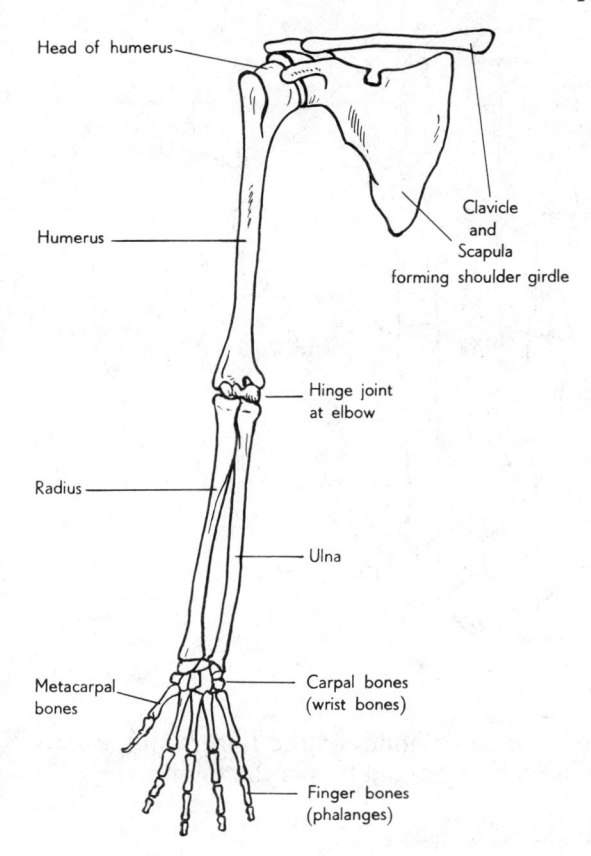

Fig. 21.9 Bones of the shoulder girdle and upper limb.

The forearm consists of two bones, the *radius,* on the thumb side of the arm, and the *ulna,* on the little finger side. At the top of the *radius* is a cup-like depression into which the lower end of the humerus fits to form the elbow joint. The point of the elbow is the upper end of the *ulna.* When the hand is turned, the lower end of the radius revolves round the ulna, forming a pivot joint.

The *wrist* is composed of eight small bones arranged in two rows of four which are called the *carpals.* Each one is capable of a slight gliding motion giving flexibility to the wrist.

The hand has five bones called the *metacarpals.* They form the framework of the palm of the hand and articulate with the bones of the fingers and thumb.

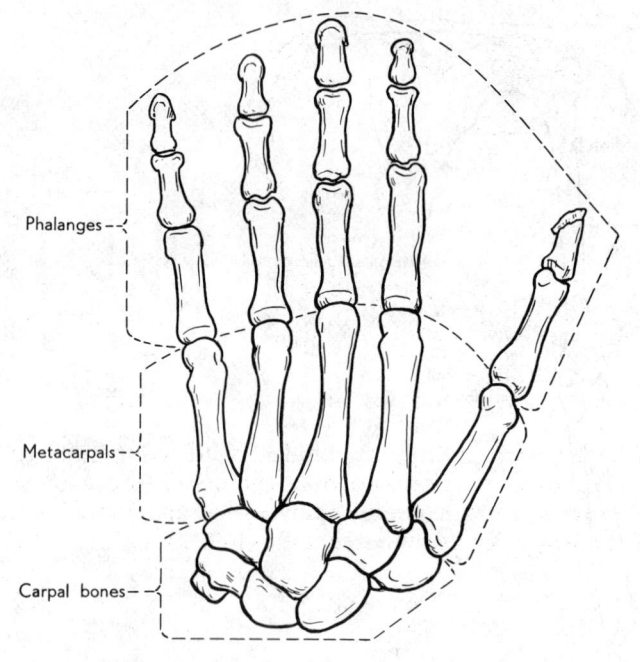

Fig. 21.10 Bones of the hand.

The *phalanges* are the short bones of the fingers and thumb (Fig. 21.10), three in each finger and two in the thumb.

Bones of the pelvis and lower limbs

The pelvic bones, together with the sacrum at the back, support the abdominal and pelvic organs and provide the deep socket for the hip joint. These bones form a girdle made up of two large, flat, irregular bones called the *innominate* bones, which articulate at the back with the sacrum and are joined in front by cartilage. The broad, upper part of each innominate bone is the *ilium*. The lower portion which supports the body when seated is the *ischium*. In the front is the *pubic bone*. On the outer side of each innominate bone is a deep, cup-like depression called the *acetabulum* into which the head of the femur fits to form the ball and socket joint of the hip (Fig. 21.11).

Bones of the leg
The *femur*, or thigh bone, is the longest bone in the body, extending from the hip joint to the knee. It is made up of a

The skeleton 187

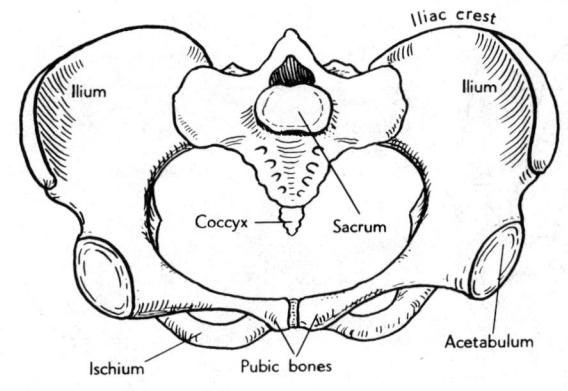

Fig. 21.11 The pelvis.

long, strong shaft, with an upper rounded head, connected to the shaft by a narrower portion known as the neck. At the lower end of the femur are two rounded ends which articulate with the bones of the lower leg at the knee joint (Fig. 21.12).

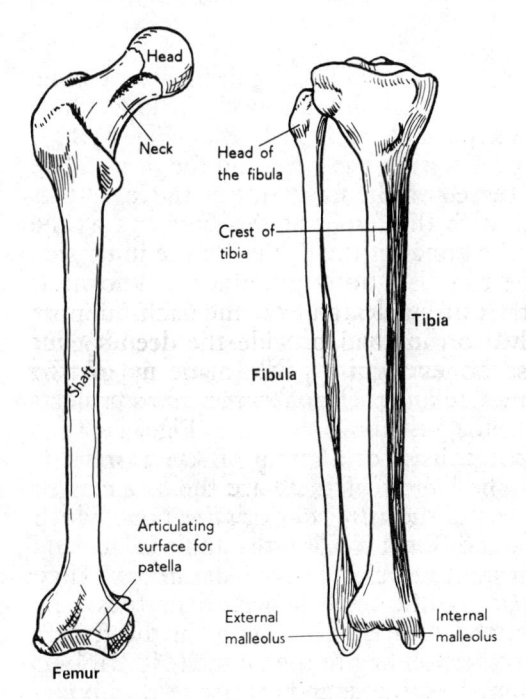

Fig. 21.12 Bones of the leg.

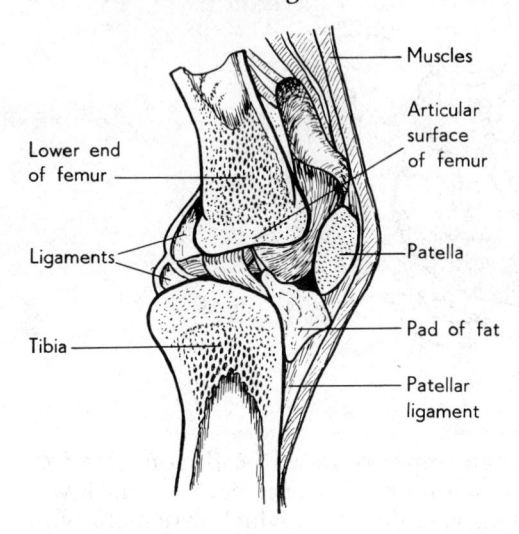

Fig. 21.13 Knee joint.

The *patella,* or knee-cap, is a small, triangular plate of bone enclosed in a fibrous capsule. It is situated over the knee joint, giving protection, and is kept in place by ligaments (Fig, 21.13).

The bones of the lower leg are the *tibia* and the *fibula.* The *tibia,* or shin bone, is situated on the inner side of the leg. At its upper end it articulates with the femur at the knee and at the lower end it joins with the bones of the ankle. On the inner side of the lower end of the tibia is a bony prominence, known as the *inner malleolus.* This can be clearly seen and felt under the skin. The *fibula* is joined to the tibia at its upper extremity but does not form part of the knee joint. The lower end of the fibula forms part of the ankle joint. The *outer malleolus* projects on the outer side of the fibula, just above the ankle (Fig. 21.12).

The bones of the foot consist of a group of seven irregular tarsal, or ankle, bones. The largest of these are the *os calcis* or *calcaneum,* the heel bone and the *astragalus* or *talus* bone which articulates with the tibia and fibula to form the ankle joint.

The bones of the instep are called the *metatarsals.* They articulate with the *phalanges,* the small bones of the toes. The number of phalanges in the toes is the same as in the fingers and thumbs. the big toe corresponding to the thumb (Fig. 21.14).

The foot is arched both lengthwise and crosswise to support the weight of the body and give springiness of movement. The

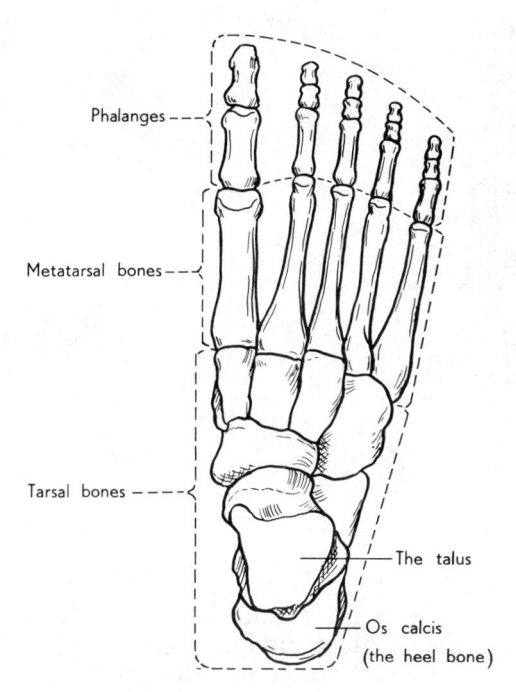

Fig. 21.14 Bones of the foot.

arches are supported by powerful ligaments. If the ligaments become stretched, the arches collapse and the condition known as flat foot results.

Joints

Joints are formed by the junction of two or more bones and may be immovable or movable.

1. *Immovable.* The edge of the bones forming this kind of joint fit closely one within the other so that no movement is possible. Typical examples of immovable joints are the sutures between the bones of the cranium.

2. *Movable.* The ends of the bones in a movable joint are protected by pads of cartilage. The joint is enclosed in a fibrous capsule which is lined with synovial membrane. This smooth membrane secretes synovial fluid which acts as a lubricant, allowing ease of movement. The whole joint is strengthened and supported by ligaments.

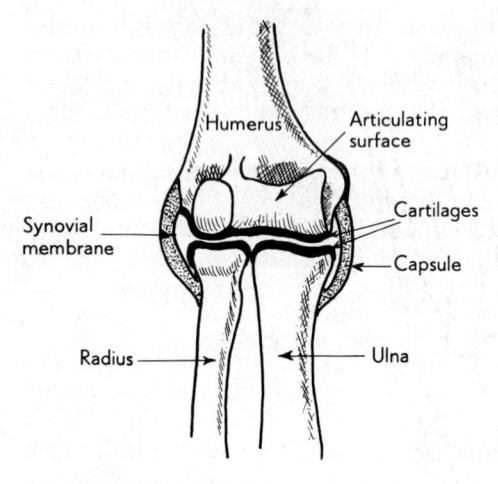

Fig. 21.15 Elbow joint.

Types of movable joints
(a) *Ball and socket joints,* where a rounded end of a long bone fits into a socket, e.g. the shoulder and hip joints.
(b) *Hinge joints,* e.g. the knee and the elbow (Figs. 21.13 and 21.15).
(c) *Gliding joints* as in the wrist and ankle.
(d) *Pivot joints,* where one bone turns on another, e.g. the atlas rotating on the axis and the radius turning on the ulna.

An imperfect movable joint is one where only slight movement is possible, as between the vertebrae.

Diseases of bones and joints

Osteoarthritis

Osteoarthritis is a disease affecting the cartilages and bone surfaces of the larger joints, as for example, the hip joint. It occurs chiefly in middle age. Symptoms include stiffness, pain and disablement.

Treatment
Treatment is the early stages includes various forms of physiotherapy such as heat, massage and controlled exercises. Drugs may be ordered for the relief of pain and a reducing diet where the patient is grossly overweight. Surgical treatment is sometimes

carried out, either by *arthrodesis*, by which the joint is immobilized and rendered permanently stiff, or by *cup arthroplasty* in which a cup-like attachment made of a specially hardened substance is fitted over the diseased and roughened bone. This provides a smooth surface, allowing the bone to move easily in its socket with consequent reduction of pain. During convalescence the patient is given graduated exercises and encouraged to walk again. The operation of total hip replacement now helps may of these patients lead a normal life again.

Rheumatoid arthritis
Rheumatoid arthritis is a progressive disease affecting the small joints of the hands in the first instance, Later, other joints of the arms or legs, and in some cases, the pelvis or the spine may become affected. The joints become stiff and very painful with wasting of the small muscles, leading to deformity, especially of the hands and feet.

Nursing care
When in bed, the patient is firmly supported with pillows, a foot rest to prevent further deformity of the feet and a large bed cradle to take the weight of the bed-clothes. A light, nourishing diet should be given. Strict attention must be paid to the care and cleanliness of the skin, especially over the pressure areas. When making the bed or carrying out nursing procedures, the patient should be handled as gently as possible, because movement usually causes acute pain.

Gout

Gout is a disease in which too much uric acid accumulates in the blood, with the result that deposits of a chalk-like substance collect in and around the joints. It occurs frequently in men of middle age. The joint of the big toe is most commonly affected, but other joints of the arms and legs may also become painful. Signs and symptoms are acute pain in the joint, redness, swelling, pyrexia and irritability.

Treatment
In the acute stage the painful joints are wrapped in cotton wool for warmth, raised on pillows and covered with a cradle to prevent pressure on the painful area. Care must be taken when moving the patient to avoid unnecessary pain. Extra fluids

should be given to prevent deposits in the kidneys. During an attack, drugs such as Phenylbutazone and Indomethacin are given. Between attacks, drugs which increase the excretion of uric acid or block its production may be prescribed. Examples of these are Probenecid and Allopurinol.

Osteomyletis

Osteomyelitis is inflammation of cancellous bone, caused by infection by staphylococcus (see p. 126). This gives rise to the formation of pus underneath the periosteum. The disease may occur as a result of tuberculosis, venereal disease or after bone injury or by blood-borne infection. Symptoms are extreme pain and tenderness over the affected area. Operative measures are usually necessary to release and drain the pus underlying the periosteum. The affected limb must be rested and antibiotics are usually prescribed in large doses.

Rickets

Rickets is a disorder of nutrition due to a lack of vitamin D in the diet (see p. 91). The disease usually affects children between the ages of 6 months and 2 years, who have been artificially fed and who live in poor conditions. At the onset the child becomes restless and irritable, with loss of appetite, vomiting, and diarrhoea. Bronchitis or convulsions may follow. The bones become soft and easily bent, giving rise to deformities. The long bones of the lower limbs often become bowed, the head has a square appearance and the fontanelles are late in closing. The sternum may grow forward producing a 'pigeon chest', and the pelvis or spine may also be deformed.

Treatment
Treatment of the deformed bones is carried out by orthopaedic or operative measures. General treatment includes a nourishing diet with a daily dose of vitamin D (see p. 91). Sunshine and fresh air are important to the progress of the patient.

Prolapsed intervertebral disc (PID).

This is a condition in which one of the intervertebral cartilages (p. 179) becomes displaced, causing acute pain in the back, loss of movement and difficulty in standing upright.

Treatment
The patient is nursed flat on a firm mattress. Traction may be applied by weights attached to the lower part of the body. In persistent cases the affected disc may be removed by surgery, but this is carried out only when other methods have proved unsuccessful.

Synovitis

Synovitis is inflammation of the synovial membrane lining a joint. The amount of synovial fluid secreted is increased and the joint becomes swollen, red, painful and difficult to move.

Treatment
The affected joint is rested by splinting. Cold or evaporating compresses may be ordered (see p. 76), followed by physiotherapy. Where the swelling persists the doctor may withdraw fluid by aspiration.

Injuries to bones and joints

Fractures

A *fracture* is a break or crack in a bone, which may occur as a result of disease, old age or injury by force or violence.

Where bone is diseased a fracture may occur as a result of changes in the formation of bone tissue. In old age the bones become brittle and easily broken. Force may be applied directly or indirectly.

1. *Direct force.* The bone breaks at the spot on which the blow falls.

2. *Indirect force.* The bone breaks at some distance from the point of impact, e.g. fracture of the spine or pelvis after falling or jumping from a height and landing on the feet.

3. *Muscular force.* A bone may be fractured by the sudden, violent contraction of the muscles attached to it, e.g. the patella may break when the knee joint is straightened forcibly to avoid falling backwards.

Types of fracture
1. *Simple* or *closed fracture*, when there is no wound leading down to the broken bone (Fig. 21.16).
2. *Compound* or *open*, when an open wound communicates

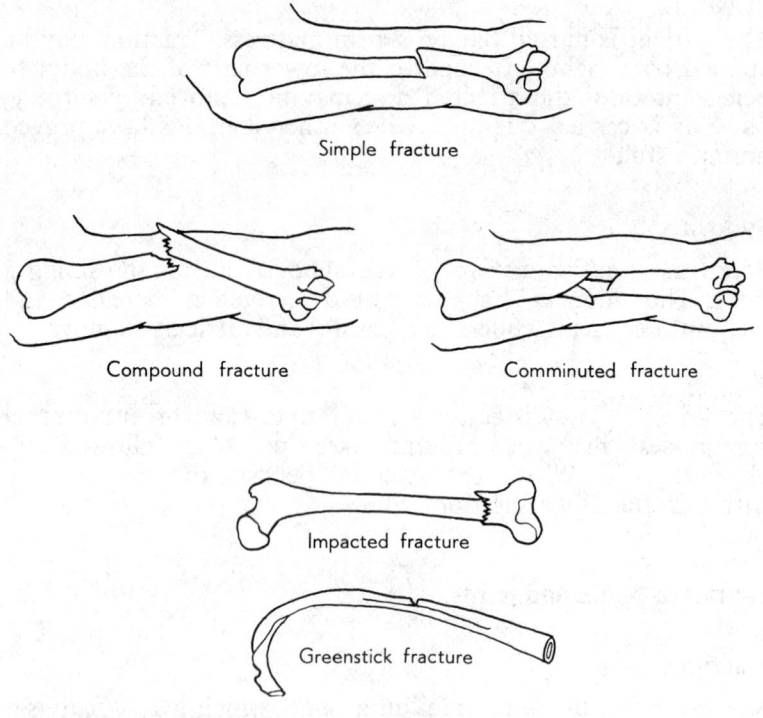

Fig. 21.16 Fractures.

with fractured bone or the broken ends of the bone pierce the skin (Fig. 21.16).

3. *Complicated fracture,* when there is injury to some internal structure or organ such as the brain, lungs, large blood vessel, or spinal cord (Fig. 21.17).

4. *Multiple fracture,* when the bone is broken in several *places.*

5. *Comminuted,* when a section of bone is broken into several *pieces* (Fig 21.16).

6. *impacted fracture,* when the broken ends are driven one into the other (Fig. 21.16).

7. *Depressed fracture,* when the broken part of the bone is driven inwards, as in a fractured skull (Fig. 21.18).

8. *Greenstick fracture* occurs in children before the bones have become hardened. The bone cracks and bends without breaking completely through (Fig 21.16).

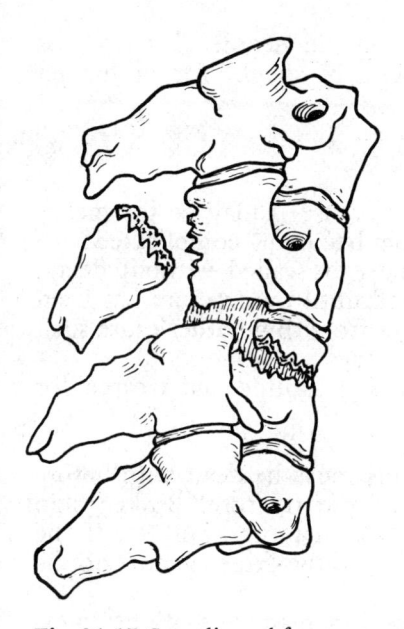

Fig. 21.17 Complicated fracture.

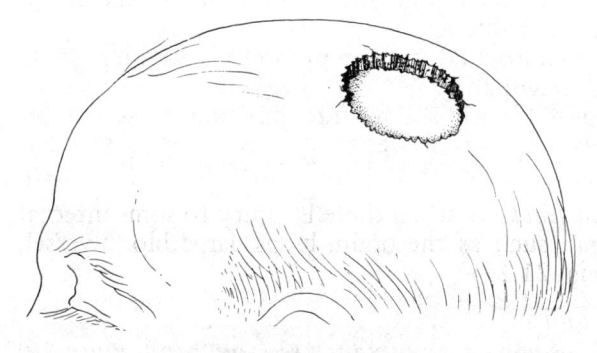

Fig. 21.18 Depressed fracture of the skull.

General signs and symptoms of fracture
 1. Pain and tenderness at, or over, the fractured area.
 2. Swelling.
 3. Loss of movement.
 4. Discoloration and bruising.
 5. Deformity of the limb.
 6. Unnatural movement at the site of the fracture.

7. Grating of the bone ends may be heard. This is called *crepitus* and must not be deliberately sought for or further injury may result.

8. Shock.

General treatment of fractures

First aid treatment is important because it may be the means of preventing a simple fracture from becoming complicated.

A doctor or an ambulance must be called without delay.

The casualty must not be moved until the fracture has been immobilized, unless there is danger from some other cause such as fire, flood, traffic or falling masonry.

The patient must be comforted, reassured and treated for shock (see p. 233).

Clothing must not be removed.

Haemorrhage and severe wounds must be dealt with before proceeding with the treatment of the fracture. Broken skin should be covered with the cleanest material available. If the wound is over the site of the fracture, the dressing must not be bandaged into place.

Splints should be applied in such a manner that the joints above and below the fracture are rendered immovable. A fractured arm may be bandaged to the chest and a broken leg may be tied to the opposite leg.

Splints may be improvised with an umbrella, a walking-stick or a thickly rolled newspaper.

Bandages used to fasten splints into position must not be applied too tightly and never over the site of a fracture. They should be fastened one above and one below the broken part of the bone.

Special fractures

Fracture of the skull

The casualty is usually unconscious, so the head must be turned to one side to prevent the tongue falling backwards over the trachea and causing asphyxia. If the breathing is noisy (sterorous) and bubbling the patient should be turned into the semi-prone position (see Fig. 26.1) and watched closely. If the base of the skull is fractured, blood and fluid may escape from the ears. On no account must any attempt be made to plug or clean the ears. The head should be turned with the affected ear on the lower side with a clean handkerchief or dressing placed underneath.

Nursing care In hospital the patient will be placed flat in bed with the head to one side in a quiet, darkened room, because noise and bright lights are a source of irritation to a patient suffering from head injuries.

The temperature is recorded every four hours and the pulse half-hourly, special note being made of the rate, rhythm and volume of the pulse (see p. 26).

Where there is compression and irritation of the brain due to head injury, the pupil of one or both eyes may become fixed and dilated. Constant and careful observation must be made for any signs of change in the size of the pupils and, if seen, must be reported without delay.

The patient should be kept warm but not overheated.

Cold compresses or ice bags may be ordered to be placed round the head.

Watch must be kept on the abdomen for any signs of distension due to retention of urine, or retention with incontinence (see p. 79).

The position of the patient should be changed at regular intervals and all pressure areas treated. If the patient is left too long in the recumbent position hypostatic pneumonia may intervene (see p. 54).

Fracture of the spine
All injuries to the spine must be regarded as serious. Fracture of a vertebra may involve the spinal cord, resulting in paralysis below the site of the fracture. In the first-aid treatment of a fractured spine the patient should not be moved until skilled help arrives, then covered with a blanket for warmth. The legs should be tied together, with pads placed between the thighs, knees and ankles. When lifting the casualty the spine must be kept rigid. The head should be held firmly so that it does not turn in any direction. Several people are required to lift the patient. This is done by working a blanket gently and carefully under him. The sides of the blanket are then rolled close to the body and used to lift the casualty on to a stretcher. At least four helpers are required to carry out this movement efficiently.

Nursing care in hospital In the first instance, the patient will be placed flat in a fracture bed made up with full-length fracture boards. A small pillow will be required to place underneath the small of the back and a foot rest to prevent foot drop. Later the patient may be nursed in the prone position (face downwards). In this case a pillow is placed under the chest, one under the thighs and a small pillow or sandbag under the ankles to keep the toes clear of the mattress. A special Stryker frame is usually used to nurse patients with serious spinal injuries.

Frequent attention to all pressure areas is important. Strict watch must be kept for any soreness or reddening of the skin. Enforced immobility and loss of sensation of the skin result in the rapid development of pressure sores.

Observation must be kept on the abdomen for signs of retention or of incontinence of urine and, these must be reported without delay.

When there is any degree of abdominal paralysis the patient may be constipated and regular enemas may be ordered to maintain bowel action. Olive-oil enemas are commonly given in such instances.

Extreme care must be taken when moving a patient with a fractured spine. Three nurses are required to do this to support the patient at the shoulders, the pelvis and the knees. Movements should be made in unison, keeping the patient's spine rigid.

Fracture of the clavicle
The arm on the injured side must be supported. A pad should be placed under the axilla over the clothing, the arm flexed across the chest and bandaged into postion. The elbow should be placed in a sling.

Fracture of the wrist (Colles' fracture)
This is a fracture of the lower end of the radius and commonly occurs as a result of falling on the outstretched hand.

Fracture of the ankle (Pott's fracture)
This is a fracture dislocation of the ankle involving the lower end of the fibula and the internal malleolus of the tibia.

Dislocation and sprains

A *dislocation* is a displacement of one or more bones at a joint. Those most frequently dislocated are the shoulder, thumb, fingers and the lower jaw.

A *sprain* is the tearing or wrenching of the ligaments and tissues round a joint. A firm bandage should be applied. Cold applications may be ordered to reduce swelling.

Repair of a fracture

In a simple fracture the broken ends of the bone are sealed by a clot of blood. This is gradually replaced by a soft tissue into which bone cells and calcium are laid down to form a solid, bony mass round fracture, called a *callus*. The callus eventually develops into new bone.

Application of plaster of Paris
Requirements
    Plaster bandages of various sizes.
    Plaster slab.
    Plaster knife.
    Plaster shears/spreader/saw, as necessary.
    Scissors
    Stockinet.
    Wool bandages.
    Bucket of tepid water.
    Plaster apron.
    Waterproof for bed.
    Waterproof for floor.
Additional requirements
    Equipment for shaving limb as necessary.
    Equipment for washing and drying limb.
    Talcum powder.
Method
Unless injured, the limb is shaved and then washed and dried. A light dusting of talcum powder is applied. Stockinet is applied, leaving extra at each end. The plaster bandages are immersed, one at a time, in the water until bubbling stops. They are squeezed to remove excess water before being handed to the operator. When the final layer is being applied, the ends of the stockinet are turned down and incorporated in the plaster. This avoids any rough edges rubbing the skin.
After Care
The plaster sets as it is put on, but takes twenty-four hours or longer to dry, depending on its size and thickness. During this time the limb is kept elevated and the extremities watched closely for any signs of blueness, coldness or loss of sensation. Any of these may indicate that the plaster cast is too tight and such an observation should be reported immediately.

Skin traction (Fig. 21.19)
This is a means of applying extension to a limb. Elastoplast

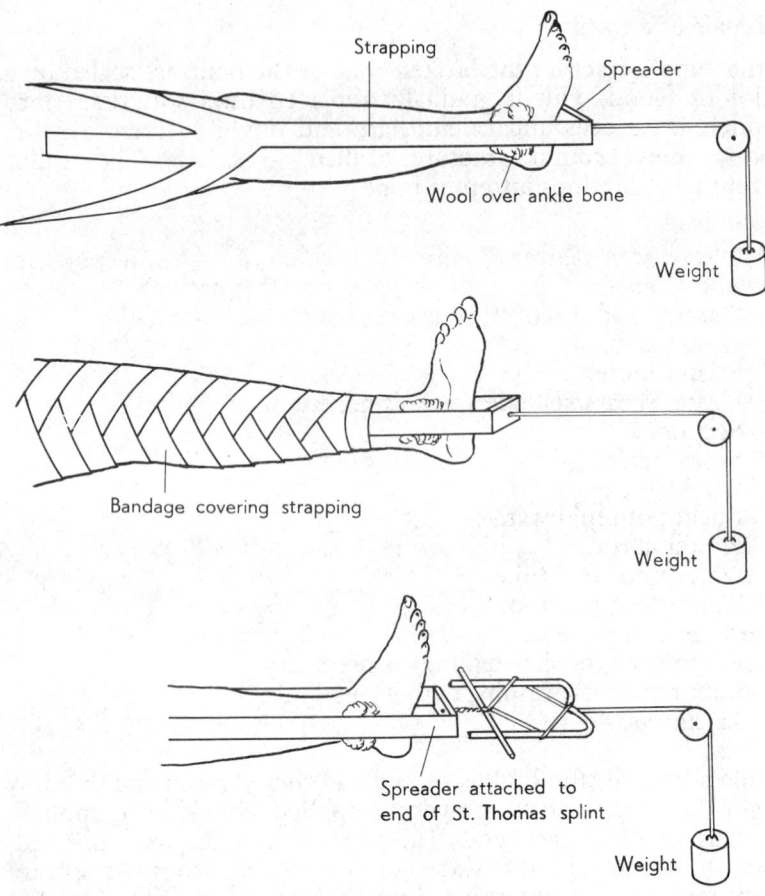

Fig. 21.19 Method of applying skin traction.

is applied to the affected limb and is connected at its lower end to a spreader and traction cord with weights attached. Skin traction kits are available, incorporating elastoplast, spreader and cord. The lower end is lined with foam to protect the malleoli.

Requirements
 Skin traction kit.
 Weights.
 Pulley and bed attachment.
 Crepe bandage, 10 cm width.
 Tincture of benzoin compound spray.

Additional requirements
  Equipment for shaving limb.
  Equipment for washing limb.
  Bed elevator, if necessary.
  Fracture board placed under mattress.

Before skin traction is applied, the skin over the area to which the strapping is to be applied must be washed with soap and water and shaved if necessary. Tincture of benzoin compound is applied to the area, which will be covered with adhesive. During the following days the patient should be watched for any signs of soreness or redness of the surrounding skin. Complaints of pain or discomfort made by the patient should be reported to the ward sister. Patients who are allergic to elastoplast may have ventfoam traction applied.

22
The reproductive system

Male reproductive organs (Fig. 22.1)

The testes are two glands situated in the scrotum, the pouch-like structure outside the body. The male reproductive cells, called spermatozoa, are produced in the testes. These glands are developed in the abdomen before birth, passing down into the scrotum at the eighth month of intra-uterine life. Where a testicle does not pass into the scrotum (undescended testicle), the condition is usually corrected by operation.

Inflammation of a testicle is known as *orchitis.*

The seminal vesicle is a small sac near the bladder, in which seminal fluid is stored.

The epididymis connects the testes with the seminal duct.

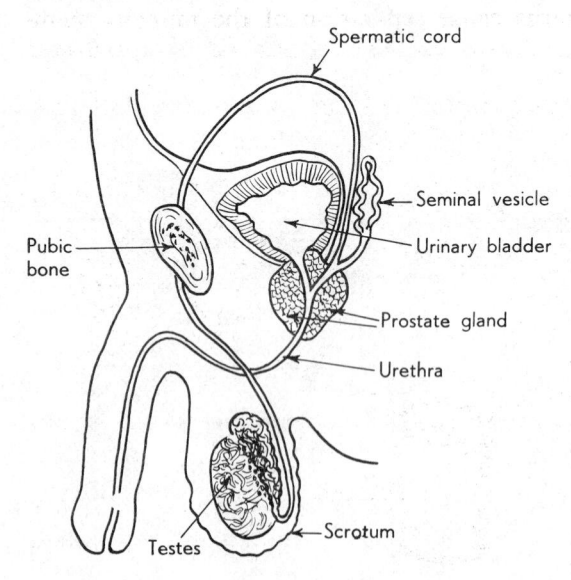

Fig. 22.1 Male reproductive organs.

The penis is the external organ connected to various internal structures concerned with reproduction. The urethra passes through the centre of the penis.

The prostate gland surrounds the urethra, where it joins with the neck of the bladder. After middle age, this gland may become enlarged and block the urethra, causing obstruction to the outflow of urine, with subsequent abdominal distension. In such cases, surgical removal of the gland may become necessary (prostatectomy).

Female reproductive organs (Fig. 22.2)

These organs are situated in the pelvic cavity. They are the uterus, the Fallopian tubes, the ovaries and the vagina. The vulva is the term used to describe the external genital organs and includes the opening of the urethra.

The uterus is a hollow, pear-shaped organ normally measuring 7.5 cm (3 in) in length, 5 cm in width and about 2.5 cm in thickness. It is kept in place by strong ligaments. The muscular wall of the uterus is immensely powerful and elastic and can be sufficiently extended to contain an infant before birth. The uterus is lined with mucous membrane, well supplied with blood vessels. During menstruation, the strong muscular contractions of the uterus cause separation of the mucous membrane and some bleeding occurs. The upper part of the uterus

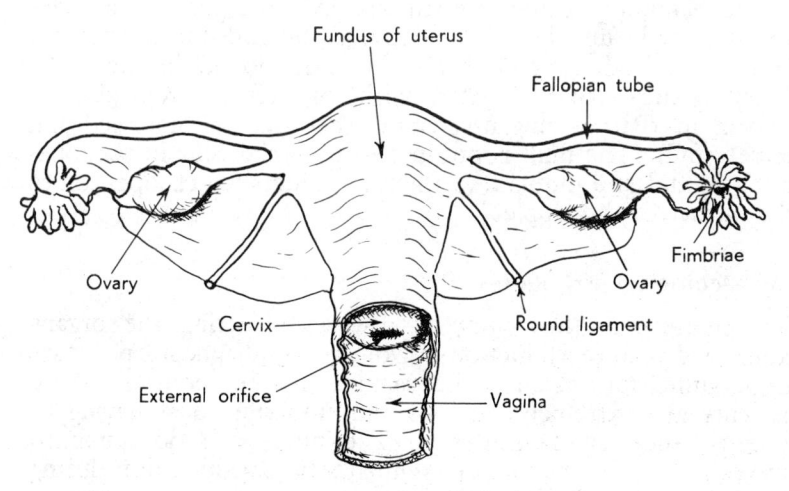

Fig. 22.2 Female reproductive organs.

is known as the body and the lower part is the *cervix,* or neck, which opens into the vagina.

The Fallopian tubes are situated one on each side of the body of the uterus. They are about 10 cm long and are supported in a wide, double fold of peritoneum known as the *broad ligament.* At their inner ends the Fallopian tubes open into the uterus. Their outer ends have a fringed opening through which the ova, or egg cells, enter. The Fallopian tubes are lined with ciliated epithelium which sweeps the ova along to the uterus (see p. 151).

The ovaries are placed one beneath each Fallopian tube. They are organs containing special cells which produce the ova. They also produce certain homones which control their activities and those of the uterus.

Every twenty-eight days, after puberty, the ova burst out of the ovaries and are swept along the Fallopian tubes to the uterus to be discharged during menstruation. When fertilization of an ovum takes place, the united cells are not discharged, but attach themsleves to the membrane lining of the uterus. From the blood vessels of this membrane the cells take nourishment and begin to grow and multiply. This is the beginning of pregnancy and a new life.

The vagina is the canal lined with mucous membrane, leading from outside the body to the uterine cervix.

The perineum is the band of tissues covered with skin situated between the external genital organs and the anus.

The mammary glands are situated over the pectoral muscles and are made up of fat, connective tissue and ducts. They are present in both sexes but remain undeveloped in the male. These glands are associated with the female reproductive system in that, during pregnancy, they become enlarged and secrete milk. The milk is produced by special cells in the lobes of the gland and drains into the many ducts which open on to the surface of the nipple.

Gynaecological procedures

Gynaecology is the study of diseases affecting the organs concerned with reproduction in women. For diagnostic purposes an examination through the vagina may be required. Many patients are extremely nervous and embarrassed at having to undergo such an examination. The nurse can do much to overcome this by tactful and sympathetic consideration during the preparation and examination of the patient. The utmost

The reproductive system

privacy must be maintained. Screens should be drawn round the bed and the bedding arranged in such a manner that there is no undue exposure of the patient. A sheet should be draped over the knees and the chest covered with a blanket. Before a vaginal examination, the bladder and rectum should be emptied and the external genitals and perineum cleansed. A folded dressing towel may be placed over the vulva to be removed on the arrival of the doctor. The patient may be placed in the recumbent, dorsal, left lateral or Sim's position, according to the wishes of the doctor.

The nurse must stay with the patient during a vaginal examination.

Tray for vaginal examination
Pack containing:
   sterile swabs;
   gallipot;
   sterile gloves;
   antibacterial cream;
   cleansing lotion;
   vaginal speculae;
   swab-holding forceps;
   blanket to cover patient's upper body;
In addition:
   anglepoise lamp;
   culture swabs;   } as necessary
   specimen containers.

23
Care of the elderly and chronically ill patient

Geriatric nursing

The term geriatric means the study and medical treatment of infirmities and diseases of elderly people. The chief aim of geriatric nursing is to help these patients regain their health and independence wherever possible.

Some years ago it was thought that frail old people should stay in bed and they were encouraged to do so, with the result that they rapidly became helpless and bedridden. Their physical needs were provided for, but little or no importance was attached to mental welfare, now considered to be an important aspect in the treatment, recovery and rehabilitation of the elderly patient.

These patients have lived active and useful lives. Some have brought up large families and most of them have had much the same interests as those of the nurses now caring for them. Many are admitted to hospital in their later years ill or neglected through no fault of their own. Some, whose relatives and friends have gone away or have died, have lived alone too long and have become depressed and lethargic, if not actually unhappy.

The average geriatric patient is in need of sympathy and understanding, and kindly, courteous nurses can, by their attitude, contribute a great deal to the recovery and eventual rehabilitation of the patient.

Where behaviour difficulties arise, the nurse should on no account show impatience or argue with elderly patients, nor force them to do anything against their will. This results only in distress on both sides and may retard the progress of the patient. Tact and gentle persuasion are usually sufficient to overcome any reluctance on the part of patients to do that which is required of them.

Those who can no longer think for themselves are as helpless as small children and need the same careful observation and attention. Many are nursed in beds fitted with protective cot sides, to prevent them falling or getting out of bed. When the patient is not receiving attention, these cot sides must be locked into position at all times to avoid the risk of accidents. Nothing should be left within reach of a confused patient with which injury might be inflicted, such as water jugs, glasses, table knives and forks or instruments of any kind.

Nursing care
Where possible, geriatric patients are nursed in the upright position to assist breathing and to lessen the risk of hypostatic pneumonia (see p. 54). The circulation tends to be poor in old age and the skin is often dry and easily broken. In the prevention of bed-sores strict observation must be given to all pressure areas, which should be treated four-hourly or more often where necessary. It must be remembered that pressure sores may also occur as a result of sitting in a chair for too long a period.

Where the physical condition permits, the patient should be allowed to take a bath in the bathroom at least once a week, but if too frail to manage this alone, two nurses will be required to lift the patient in and out of the bath. Where shower baths are in use, the patient must be given firm support whilst standing and a seat provided for safety and to give confidence. An elderly patient taking a shower must not be left alone for even a moment.

A non-slip bath mat should be placed at the side of the bath and another in the bottom of the bath to prevent the patient from slipping on the wet surfaces. A chair covered with a bath towel should be placed near the bath so that the patient can sit comfortably whilst being dried. The door of the bathroom must not be locked and the patient should not be left alone in the bathroom for any length of time in case of accidental injury.

After the bath the toe- and finger nails should be trimmed if the patient is unable to do this. The hair should be washed weekly if possible and, for female patients, should be well brushed and combed and arranged as attractively as possible.

The mouth should receive frequent attention, especially where the patient is unable to clean the teeth. Dentures should be removed for cleansing after each meal and should be scrubbed thoroughly under running water, using the patient's toothbrush. A gauze swab can be used when removing the dentures of helpless patients.

Diet
A nourishing well-balanced diet will be ordered according to

the condition of the patient. Small quantities should be served and the patient encouraged to eat all or most of the food given her. If for any reason food or drink is refused, the nurse should report the matter to the ward sister, because nourishment is important in the care and recovery of the aged. For details of feeding helpless patients see page 102.

Incontinence
Incontinence in the elderly is not deliberate. In old age the muscles controlling the bladder become weak and the patient may have difficulty in retaining urine, even for a short time. A bed-pan or urinal should be given as soon as requested. Most elderly patients suffer mental distress from their incontinence, although unable to express their anxiety. The patient should be reassured and treated with kindness to alleviate any distress which may be felt.

Ambulation
Ambulation means that the patient can get out of bed and move around the ward. Where the physical condition allows, geriatric patients are encouraged to do as much for themselves as possible. Movement stimulates the circulation, the digestion of foods, good muscle tone, prevents the joints from becoming stiff, and revives interest in the activities of the ward and in other people. The patient should be encouraged to dress as fully as possible, including shoes and stockings and to take pride in the appearance. This assists in maintaining self-respect and is an advance towards eventual rehabilitation. For those patients who can sit only in a chair, comfort should be the first consideration. The chair should have arm rests and a high back to give adequate support. A rug or coloured blanket should be arranged across the seat of the chair so that the patient sits on the centre of the rug and the ends can then be folded over the legs and knees, and tucked firmly in at the sides. Where there is risk of incontinence, an incontinence pad may be placed over the rug on the seat of the chair. A cushion or pillow should be placed at the back of the head so that it is firmly supported in an upright position and the feet should rest firmly on the floor or on a footstool. When the patient is comfortably settled in the chair, the nurse should make sure that anything the patient may need is within easy reach so that no attempt will be made to stand or walk unaided.

The chronically ill patient

A chronic disease is one where progress is slow and is therefore of long duration. Examples are paralysis due to brain or spinal injuries or disease, Parkinson's disease, chronic affections of the heart or lungs and multiple sclerosis.

Chronic disease may affect people of all ages and often brings a sense of frustration and hopelessness with the fear of becoming unwanted and a burden to others. The attitude of the nurse towards these patients should be one of quiet cheerfulness, with a lively interest in their progress and welfare. They should be encouraged to do as much as possible for themselves, however long a time this may take, and may require as much patience on the part of the nurse as that of the patient who should not be hurried. Praise given where such attempts are made will give confidence and courage to continue their efforts.

Occupational therapy, in which hands and brain are brought into action, is invaluable in rousing the interest of the patient and making life a little happier. Such occupations as knitting, embroidery, making rugs, lampshades or soft toys, reading or painting can all be profitably employed. Games such as chess, cards or dominoes will also provide diversion, especially amongst male patients. Newspapers, books and periodicals should be made available for those patients who can read, in order to maintain interest in events taking place outside the hospital.

Companionship is important to the chronically sick patient and many of them, particularly the elderly, delight in talking about their lives and their families. The nurse should be prepared to listen and show an intelligent interest in what they have to say. In this way a greater insight into the personal problems and anxieties of individual patients may be obtained, creating an invaluable bond of sympathy and understanding between nurse and patient.

24
Burns, diabetes, neoplasms, tuberculosis, venereal diseases, last offices

Burns

Burns may be caused by dry heat, moist heat (scalds), electricity, chemicals, x-rays or radio-active substances, The severity of a burn is assessed according to the depth of tissue injured, as follows.

Superficial burn with *partial skin destruction* which may affect wide areas of skin with redness and blistering. These burns usually heal without complications, provided infection is prevented. Where blistering is extensive, large quantities of serum escape from the underlying tissues resulting in a serious loss of body fluids and salts, with accompanying shock.

Deep burn with *full thickness destruction* of tissue. In such cases treatment will depend on the depth and extent of the burn. Skin grafting may become necessary to reduce the risk of contraction and deformity.

All burns should be considered dangerous to life, especially where large areas of body are involved and in children and old people.

General treatment of burns

Superficial burns may be gently irrigated with cold water to lessen the initial pain and should then be covered with a clean dry towel or dressing. Blisters must be left intact until seen by the doctor who will give instructions as to their treatment.

Patients suffering from more severe burns are usually given morphia on admission to counteract shock and relieve pain. Extensive dressings may be carried out under a general anaesthetic and routine injections of antibiotics may be ordered to prevent infection.

Where possible, the patient should be nursed in the upright position to avoid risk of pneumonia.

Burns may be treated in the open or closed method, but in

either instance gowns and masks must be worn by all staff attending the patient.

In the *open* or *exposed* method, the patient, usually a child, is nursed in a cubicle kept at a temperature of 24° to 27°C (or 75° to 80°F). The burned areas are protected by a bed cradle and exposed to the air.

A crust forms over the burn and protects the underlying tissues from infection. This crust separates in about fourteen to twenty-one days, but if progress is not then satisfactory, skin grafting may be carried out by the surgeon. Where a joint is involved, the limb must not remain flexed or permanent deformity may result. A high protein diet with plenty of fluids is given, but where the patient is severely ill, fluids are introduced intravenously. A strict fluid chart must be kept in order to check the loss of body fluids from damaged tissues.

In the *closed* method, dressings are used with strict aseptic precautions according to instructions given by the doctor.

Complications of burns

These include shock, pneumonia or acute bronchitis, sepsis and toxaemia, deformity, loss of movement, nephritis or renal failure.

For emergency treatment of burns, see page 244.

Diabetes mellitus

Special groups of cells in the pancreas, known as the islets of Langerhans, secrete a substance called *insulin* which serves to balance the amount of sugar in the bloodstream. Failure of these cells to function efficiently results in diabetes mellitus. This is a condition in which glucose, normally stored in the liver as glycogen, accumulates in the blood, eventually appearing in the urine.

Overweight people may develop signs of diabetes during middle age. Such patients may be producing insulin in the pancreas, but for some unknown reason, excess fat prevents the efficient action of insulin. In such cases the correct diet will often restore the balance of blood sugar to normal. The diabetic diet aims at providing the maximum amount of nourishment required by the body without excess sugar. This is achieved by giving plenty of protein, green vegetables and vitamins, while restricting the amount of carbohydrates and fats.

Diabetes in young people may develop where the islets of

Langerhans do not function and no insulin in manufactured. It is then necessary to introduce insulin by artificial means to avoid hyperglycaemia and ketosis (see p. 214). Heredity plays some part in the incidence of diabetes. A tendency to contract the disease may occur and reoccur in families.

The nurse takes an important part in the care and progress of the diabetic patient, being responsible for giving the correct diet, the correct dosage of insulin, the daily testing of urine, for weighing the patient at regular intervals, for keeping accurate records of all treatment and investigations, and for advising and reassuring the patient. Extreme care must be taken of the skin, in the prevention of bed sores, and when trimming the toe- or fingernails. Broken skin in the diabetic is difficult and slow to heal. In some cases there is loss of feeling, especially of the feet, so that the patient is unaware of the heat, pain or soreness of the skin. Where bed cradles are in use, they should be placed in such a position that the feet and toes do not come into contact with the bars of the cradle. The most efficient types of cradles are those which fit underneath the mattress at the bottom or side of the bed and have no bars to cause injury to the patient's skin.

Changes in the level of the blood sugar may have an effect on the brain, resulting in confusion, obstinacy, emotional outbursts or other abnormal behaviour. Realizing this, the nurse should at all times show patience and tolerance. As treatment progresses these symptoms will disappear.

Types of insulin

1. *Soluble insulin* is given mainly in emergency. It has a rapid action but the effect lasts for about eight hours only. It is not suitable for continued treatment because injection may be needed two or three times a day. The solution is made in strengths of 20, 40 and 80 units per ml and should be clear in appearance.

2. *Protamine zinc insulin* is absorbed slowly, giving an overall effect for eighteen hours.

3. *Insulin zinc suspension semi-lente* has a rapid action after administration lasting about ten hours.

4. *Insulin zinc suspension ultra-lente* acts slowly and is effective for up to twenty hours.

5. *Insulin zinc suspension lente* is a mixture of semi-lente and ultra-lente, giving a rapid and slow action together to cover twenty-four hours.

There are now newer insulins on the market which are thought to cause less local tissue damage. These are purified beef and porcine insulins and are manufactured under such names as Actrapid, Neusulin and Neulente.

Administration of insulin

A special syringe is used which is divided into 20 'marks' per ml for the measurement of units of insulin; one mark on the syringe represents one unit of single strength soluble insulin, two units of 40 strength insulin and four units of 80 strength insulin.

Insulin is supplied in three strengths, 20, 40 and 80 units per ml. Each type of insulin is labelled in a different colour with the number of units per ml clearly marked on the label. When preparing an injection of insulin, nurses should not rely entirely on the colours of the labels but should be careful to read the name and strength of the insulin printed on the container. The injection must be checked by a State Registered nurse before administration. Insulin is given hypodermically and the sites of the injections should be widely scattered and used in rotation to prevent thickening and disfiguration of the skin. This is especially important for young people. The outer sides of the upper arms, the thighs and the skin over the abdomen may be used in turn.

For the middle-aged, overweight patients, tolbutamide (Rastinon), chlorpropamide (Diabinese) or similar tablets may be ordered for the control of diabetes. These tablets are taken by mouth in conjunction with a strict low-carbohydrate diet. They contain substances which increase the output of insulin from the pancreas. They do not contain insulin and are of no value in severe diabetes.

The diabetic at home

Before being discharged from hospital, the diabetic patient should be shown how to test urine for sugar. (For this purpose the Clinitest outfit is the simplest for home use, see p. 81). The patient should also be shown how to assemble, dismantle and sterilize the syringe and needle. Advice should be given on the care of the feet, with regular treatment by a chiropodist. The importance of regular dental care should be stressed.

Diabetic patients should carry with them at all times a card bearing their name and address, the name, address and telephone number of the private doctor or diabetic clinic being attended, the type and amount of insulin taken and the time of administration. Several cubes of sugar, glucose tablets or sweet biscuits should be carried in the handbag or pocket to be taken at the first signs of faintness or mental confusion. These are the first symptoms of hypoglycaemia (see below) and may occur if too little food is taken after an injection of insulin, or on violent or unaccustomed exercise. This should be explained to all diabetic patients so that they may guard against such an occurrence by taking, in emergency, a little sugar.

Hypoglycaemia
Hypoglycaemia, or insulin coma, means that there is too little sugar in the blood. The onset is sudden and the signs and symptoms include sweating, pallor or flushing of the face, bounding pulse, mental confusion, obstinacy and some speech disturbance. Convulsions may occur, especially in children, or unconsciousness. These symptoms are relieved by taking sugar. If the patient is unconscious, intravenous glucose may be given, usually with good effect.

Hyperglycaemia
Hyperglycaemia, or diabetic coma, is the result of too much sugar in the blood. The onset is gradual and the symptoms include loss of appetite, vomiting, abdominal pain, rapid, shallow respirations, drowsiness and lethargy, followed by unconsciousness. Large amounts of urine are passed. A distinct sweet smell of acetone can be noted in the breath and skin.

Treatment The patient is treated for shock and is kept warm without overheating, to avoid further loss of body fluids. If unconscious, the patient will be catheterized to obtain a specimen of urine to be tested for sugar, ketone bodies and albumin. A self-retaining catheter may be left in place and urine taken off at stated intervals. A strict fluid chart should be recorded. Blood specimens will be taken for blood sugar estimation and the results will also be recorded. Soluble insulin may be ordered by the doctor to be given either by intramuscular or intravenous injection, for the unconscious patient an intravenous infusion may be ordered in addition. In certain cases where the stomach is distended, a stomach washout may be ordered to evacuate the remains of any carbohydrates the patient may have taken. A nasogastric tube may be left in place for aspiration of the stomach or for feeding purposes. On recovery from the coma, the dosage of insulin can be established and regular urine testing carried out at two- to four-hourly intervals.

Neoplasms

Neoplasms are new growths which take place in the body and may be benign or malignant in character.

Benign or harmless growths are enclosed in a capsule and do not spread into the surrounding tissues, but where they increase in size they may cause pressure and become painful, necessitaing surgical treatment. Benign tumours include such growths as fibromas, lipomas or adenomas. If not treated, these benign growths may eventually become malignant.

Malignant growths are divided into two main groups, *sarcoma* and *carcinoma*.

Sarcoma

Sarcoma is less common than carcinoma and may affect bone, muscle or fibrous tissue, usually in the young patient.

Carcinoma

Carcinoma occurs in animals as well as in human beings. It is not considered to be hereditary and no race is exempt from this disease. Some forms of carcinoma can be cured by surgery, radium and radiotherapy and drugs. Other carcinomas have proved to be incurable, although research is constantly being carried out to find the cause and hence the cure for this disease. The cells of carcinoma travel in lymph and in the bloodstream, and, when established in the body, create toxins which cause severe illness and occasionally marked behaviour changes in the patient. The growth of carcinoma is not enclosed in a capsule and can infiltrate into other tissues and organs. Symptoms vary according to the organs affected, but pain rarely occurs in the early stages. It is for this reason that early diagnosis and treatment are essential.

After surgical removal of a malignant growth, secondary growths may appear some time, often years, later in another part of the body, involving the nearest lymphatic glands.

Inoperable carcinoma is a condition in which the disease is too far advanced for surgical treatment. Very little can be done beyond skilled and diligent nursing, and every possible care given for the comfort and relief of the patient.

Tuberculosis

Tuberculosis is a notifiable disease, caused by the tubercle bacillus, which invades body tissues, causing them to become inflamed, damaged or destroyed. The disease may be acute or chronic and can affect most of the body tissues. It is not considered to be hereditary, although there may be a predisposing tendency towards the disease in families. There are two types of tubercle bacillus, bovine and human.

Bovine tubercle bacillus enters the gastrointestinal tract by the drinking of infected milk. This type of tuberculosis in now almost eradicated by strict supervision of dairy herds, the production of tuberculin-tested milk and by pastuerization of all milk.

Human tubercle bacillus is spread by inhalation of the bacteria in crowded, badly ventilated rooms, by careless coughing and sneezing, in excretions from people suffering from the disease, and by spitting in public places. In the latter instance, the sputum dries and the tubercle bacilli are released to float in the air, carrying the infection to other people. These bacteria can live in dust for many months and become active when released into the air.

Tuberculosis can be divided into two main classes, *pulmonary tuberculosis* which affects the lungs and *non-pulmonary tuberculosis* affecting other structures, such as the skin and bones.

Pulmonary tuberculosis

General signs and symptoms
Debility, loss of weight, lethargy, cough, dyspnoea, copious sputum which may be bloodstained, night sweats, and in advanced cases there may be haemoptysis.

Nursing care
If admitted to hospital, the patient is isolated or barrier nursed (see p 129). Nursing care includes rest, nourishing diet, freedom from anxiety, and fresh air. The patient should be weighed each week to check the loss or gain in weight. Extreme care must be taken against the spread of infection. Paper handkerchiefs should be provided, and the patient taught to cover the mouth when coughing. The disposable handkerchiefs should be burned as soon as possible after being used. All

excreta should be disinfected before disposal and linen treated as infectious.

Preventive measures
Prevention can be effected by early investigation, good living conditions, mass x-ray, and continued observation of suspected cases and contacts, for a minimum period of two years, by the medical and health visiting staffs attached to the chest clinics; by education of the general public in cleanliness in the home, food hygiene, and advantages of fresh air and good ventilation and the extreme danger of spitting in the streets, or other public places.

Non-pulmonary tuberculosis

This type includes affections of the bones, joints, skin, glands or internal organs, other than the lungs, and may be the result of infection by the bovine tubercle bacillus. Patients with this type of tuberculosis are usually kept in care and under observation for many months.

Mantoux test
This is a skin test to find out whether a person is susceptible to tubercular infection. A minute amount of the toxin produced by the tubercle bacillus is injected under the skin. A red, raised area developing around the point of the injection indicates a positive reaction and denotes immunity. Where there is a negative reaction and no redness appears at the site of injection, this indicates that there is no resistance to tuberculosis. In such cases vaccination with BCG (bacillus Calmette-Guérin) is carried out. This is a means of preventing tuberculosis and is now a routine measure for babies born into families with a history of the disease. Nurses and medical students having a negative Mantoux test are also protected from the disease by BCG vaccination.

The Heaf test
The Heaf test is another skin test for tuberculosis. A drop of the vaccine is placed on the skin and is driven into the skin with a special 'gun' syringe. This makes several tiny punctures through which the tuberculin is absorbed.

Patch test with tuberculin jelly
The skin between the shoulder blades is cleansed with surgical

218 *Practical nursing*

spirit or acetone. A little tuberculin jelly is squeezed on to the skin, covered with Elastoplast and left for forty-eight hours. Redness or slight swelling over the area denotes a positive reaction.

A positive reaction means that at some time infection by the tubercle bacillus has occurred, which may not have resulted in active tuberculosis but has produced a certain immunity to the disease.

Venereal diseases

Syphilis and gonorrhoea are the two most common venereal diseases. Both are extremely dangerous and should be treated as early as possible. These diseases are spread by direct contact, mainly during sexual intercourse. They can also be spread by contact with articles such as sheets or towels contaminated by discharges from an infected person. Nurses should be extremely careful when attending an infected patient. Gloves should be worn to protect the hands which should be thoroughly washed after attending an infected patient. All equipment used for and by the patient should be clearly marked and kept separate from that in general use.

Syphilis

This disease may be acquired as described above or inherited from the mother, who may have been infected by the father of the child. Untreated syphilis passes through three stages, as follows.

The primary stage
The incubation period is from ten days to ten weeks. The initial lesion develops into an ulcer, called a *chancre,* and the surrounding lympathic glands become enlarged. The primary sore disappears in a few weeks.

The secondary stage
This period indicates a general infection of the whole body and may occur before or after the primary sore disappears. During this stage any of the following symptoms may appear — sore throat, ulcerated tonsils, sores in the mouth, loss of hair, a copper-coloured non-irritating rash, enlarged lymphatic glands, anaemia and soft warty masses round the anus and genital organs.

Syphilis is extremely contagious during the primary and secondary stages, In the primary stage the sore which forms at the point of inoculation by the micro-organisms is very infectious. During the secondary stage, when the whole body is infected, all secretions and discharges carry infection.

The tertiary stage
The symptoms of advanced disease may appear within two to ten years from the onset. In this last stage the disease may attack such tissues of the body as the skin and mucous membranes, causing soft swellings called gummata, or the bones, periosteum, liver or the central nervous system. The patient may die from chronic disease of the circulatory or nervous systems.

Congenital or hereditary syphilis

This may be evident soon after birth or may become apparent later in childhood. Early symptoms include wasting of the body, vesicles or pustules of the hands and feet, inflammation of the bones and especially the growing ends of bones, snuffles with profuse nasal discharge or enlargement of the liver or spleen. Later symptoms are inflammation of the cornea of the eye, a depressed bridge of the nose, giving a characteristic facial appearance, changes in the internal ear leading to deafness, notched and peg-shaped front teeth, known as Hutchinson's teeth, and nervous symptoms. Courses of treatment are repeated until the blood tests give a negative Wasserman reaction.

Congenital syphilis in the newborn may be prevented by a full course of treatment during pregnancy. Antiobiotics have been found to be effective in the treatment of the disease and are now used extensively.

Gonorrhoea

This is the venereal disease, caused by the gonococcus, which may infect the mucous membrane of any of the genital organs.

The incubation period is from two to ten days. In the male it causes a purulent discharge from the urethra (urethritis) accompanied by painful micturition. In women the cervix of the uterus and the urethra are commonly affected with a purulent discharge from the vagina.

Complications in the male include inflammation of the testes (orchitis) and stricture or obstruction of the urethra. In the female, inflammation of the Fallopian tubes may develop (salpingitis), or peritonitis or sterility. Inflammation of the joints (gonococcal arthritis) or heart disease may affect both sexes.

The chief complication affecting the newborn is inflammation of the eyes (ophthalmia neonatorum) as a result of infection contracted during birth. This is a serious condition which, if untreated, may cause blindness. Close observation is made during the first few weeks of life for any signs or redness or discharge from the eyes. Where these symptoms arise, the child is isolated, the doctor is notified and treatment commenced without delay. Irrigation of the eyes and the insertion of special eye drops may be ordered.

Preventive measures include ante-natal examination and treatment of the mother and careful cleansing of the eyelids of the baby as soon as the head is born. Specialist treatment is given by State Registered nurses for ophthalmia neonatorum.

Last offices

When signs of approaching death become evident, the relatives of the patient and the minister of religion are notified by the ward sister or deputy.

Relatives should be treated with sympathetic courtesy and quiet consideration. They may wish to stay at the bedside or they may prefer to wait in another room. If very shocked, no friend or relative should be allowed to leave the hospital until treatment is given, with full recovery. Before leaving, they should be referred to the ward sister or nurse in charge who will advise them as to the issue of the certificate of death and the collection of the patient's belongings. Nurses must not express their own opinions as to the cause of collapse or death of the patient. Any enquiries on this point must be referred to the sister, who will in turn refer them to the doctor in charge of the case.

Last offices are carried out in two stages, The first stage is undertaken as soon as possible after death has occurred and before the muscles become stiffened. This stiffening of the muscles is known as *rigor mortis* (see p. 155).

The second stage is performed about one hour later. This is the last service that the nurse is able to carry out for the patient and must be performed with the utmost reverence. Two nurses should work quietly together with no unnecessary talking between them.

First stage
The bed is stripped, leaving the top sheet over the patient and a small pillow under the head. All other equipment, such as air rings, cradles, hot-water bottles, oxygen apparatus or continuous drip stands, should be removed from the bedside.

Jewellery which the patient may be wearing should be removed, with the exception of a wedding ring. With regard to this the relatives must be consulted and their wishes carried out.

The patient's eyes are closed and the lids covered with cotton-wool swabs. A small pillow placed firmly under the chin will keep the lower jaw in the closed position without bruising the chin. The body is arranged as straight as possible with the arms at the sides and a pad of wool placed between the ankles before tying them together. The body is then covered with a sheet and left for one hour. During this time the equipment needed for the second stage is collected on a trolley.

Second stage
After the second stage has been started the nurses should not leave the bedside until the procedure is completed.

Requirements
Bowl of hot water, soap, flannels and towels.

Brush and comb and white ribbon for the female patient with long hair.

Gauze swabs.

Scissors, nail scissors. Elastoplast and waterproof plaster.

Receptacles for soiled instruments and dressings.

Clean sheets, pillow-cases and shroud, which are usually kept for this purpose only.

Two labels with the name of the patient, the ward, the date and time of death, and tapes to tie the labels to the patient's wrist and ankle.

Method The body is washed all over very thoroughly, using plenty of soap, and the finger- and toenails cut and left very clean. If there is a wound, the dressings are removed, together with any drainage tubes. The area is cleaned and covered with clean gauze swabs which are then held in place with waterproof strapping.

The patient is dressed in the gown provided. The hair is brushed and arranged neatly and as attractively as possible; the hair of a female patient may be tied with white ribbon. Metal hair grips, pins or slides must not be used.

A clean sheet is rolled underneath the patient and the soiled one removed. A second clean sheet covers the body. When everything necessary has been done, the labels are fastened securely to the wrist and ankles, the porters are notified and the body removed from the ward with as little disturbance of other patients as possible.

Personal posessions of the patient should be made into a parcel to be handed to the relatives. All valuables, including letters, pension book or documents should be listed in duplicate, checked by another nurse, parcelled separately and handed to the ward sister for safe keeping.

All equipment used by the patient, must be cleaned or disposed of without delay. Sheets and blankets are sent to the laundry, pillows are sent for fumigation where necessary. The bed is washed before being made up with fresh linen. The locker is washed inside and out. During the whole procedure the screen should remain closed round the bed and should not be removed until the clean bed and locker are in their normal places. When all equipment has been removed and everything is neat and tidy the screen may be withdrawn.

The trolley is cleaned and all bowls and instruments cleaned and sterilized immediately.

25
The normal baby

The average baby at birth weighs about 3.5 kg (7lb) and is about 50 cm (20 in) in length. The head is large, usually measuring about 32 cm (13 in) in circumference, the face is small by comparison. The eyes of most newly born babies are blue, changing in colour as they grow older.

The pulse is rapid and irregular at about 120 to 140 beats per minute, with respirations about 30 to 40 per minute.

Tears do not appear until the sixth or eighth week of life. The infant sleeps for almost twenty-four hours each day, waking only for feeding and bathing.

Sudden movements and loud noises will startle and disturb a small baby. When handling and lifting the child the movements should be quiet and gentle, but firm enough to give a feeling of security.

Clothing should be loose, light in weight and warm. Cot covers should be tucked firmly, but not tightly, under the mattress because a small baby needs to feel supported at all times.

The teeth begin to form in the gums before birth but do not erupt until after the fifth month, although the gums may become red and swollen as early as the fourth month, giving rise to signs of irritability.

The normal baby is fed every three or four hours according to the body weight. As weight gains are stabilized, feeds should be given every four hours. During the first few weeks the feeding schedule should not be too rigid. The infant should not be left to cry excessively when a feed is almost due, but should be picked up, comforted and fed. Eventually routine feeding times will become successfully established.

During the first three or four months the weight increases by about 175 g (or 6 oz) a week, after which this amount gradually lessens.

At 6 months the birth weight is doubled. The child can sit up comfortably and takes a lively interest in people, movements, colours and sounds. When teething has commenced, the two lower incisors are usually the first to be seen. At this age the infant will sleep for about sixteen hours each day. Exercise is important and the baby should be given the opportunity to kick freely. To do this the baby should be warmly dressed and put on a rug on the floor, preferably in a play pen. In hospital the child may be placed on top of the blankets in the cot. The cot sides must be securely locked in the closed position.

At one year the birth weight is trebled. The child becomes more active, can move around and can pull himself into the standing position.

The pulse rate is about 110 beats per minute, respirations about 32 per minute. The child will sleep about fourteen hours a day. During the next few months the anterior fontanelle should become gradually smaller and should be closed by 18 months.

The child in hospital

The majority of sick children cannot explain how they feel, but to the observant nurse any change in their appearance or condition is immediately apparent. Strict observation must be kept at all times and any abnormal signs or symptoms must be reported without delay to the ward sister or the deputy.

Cries
The character of a cry will indicate the cause. The normal cry is loud and usually prolonged and the infant kicks and becomes red in the face.

A low whining cry is a sign of exhaustion.

Sharp, piercing screams at intervals may indicate disease of the brain. Between the screams the child lies quietly on the back.

Loud crying whilst drawing up the legs indicates abdominal pain or discomfort.

A hoarse, whispering cry is a symptom of inflammation of the throat.

With inflammation of the lungs the child grunts but does not cry aloud because taking a deep breath causes pain.

Stools
The colour, consistency, frequency and size of the stools should be noted and reported, because they are an important guide to the progress and condition of the baby and are an indication of suitability of the type of feed the infant is having.

The stools of breast-fed babies are large and mustard coloured and those from infants fed on any form of cows' milk are a paler yellow.

Green or yellow frothy stools indicate that too much starch is being given.

Dark green stools are signs that the baby is under-fed.

Bright green stools may be due to over feeding or to some intestinal infection.

Clay or putty-coloured stools are due to excess fat in the diet.

Curds seen in a stool are a sign that the food is not being digested.

Brown stools normally occur after mixed feeding is introduced.

Sore buttocks
Constant care must be given to the skin covering the buttocks and legs of a baby to avoid the redness and soreness which may arise from wet napkins. This is especially important where the stools are abnormally loose and frequent. Napkins should be changed as soon as they become soiled, the skin washed with warm water, dried gently and thoroughly, and powdered with dusting powder. Zinc and castor oil cream or petroleum jelly may also be applied and is beneficial in protecting the skin from moisture, All folds and creases in the skin of the legs and buttocks should be powdered lightly to prevent soreness due to moisture collecting in the crevices.

Bathing a baby

Requirements
  Baby bath.
  Bath thermometer.
  Gallipot.
  Bath towel.
  Cotton-wool balls.
  Soap.
  Clinical thermometer.
  Clean clothes.
  Clean napkin.
  Hairbrush.
  Nail scissors.
  Talcum powder.
  Baby creams, as necessary.

226 Practical nursing

Pedal bin for soiled linen.
Pedal bin for soiled disposables.
Plastic apron for nurse.

Method Where possible the baby should be lifted from the cot and bathed on the lap, but everything needed for the bath should be collected and prepared before lifting the baby.

Each child should have its own towels. The nurse should wear a plastic apron covered with a flannel or towelling apron. (A separate apron should be worn for each baby.) The room must be warm and free from draught.

When preparing the bath, cold water must be run in first and hot water added until the correct temperature is reached. The temperature of the water must be checked with a bath thermometer. The water should be prepared at 41°C (or 105°F) and should be checked again before putting the baby into the bath, when it should register 38°C (or 100°F).

Before disturbing the baby, the pulse and repsirations should be counted and recorded. (The temperature is taken when the baby is undressed.)

The baby is undressed completely, except for the napkin, and wrapped firmly in a bath towel. The arms should be enclosed.

1. Swab the eyes with clean warm water using each swab once only.

2. Carefully wash and dry the face using plain water and wool swabs. The inside of the mouth, nose and ears should be left alone.

3. The infant's legs and trunk should be held under the nurse's arm with the head over the bath, supported by the hand. Thoroughly wet the scalp before applying soap. Gently massage with the hand, then rinse well, removing all traces of soap. Dry the head with a soft towel. This must be done very carefully because the anterior fontanelle is still open.

4. Unwrap the towel from the child and spread it over the lap. Remove the napkin. Cleanse the buttocks and take the rectal temperature. At this stage the baby is weighed, if necessary.

5. With the baby on the lap, make a soapy lather in the hands and apply it gently to the body of the child, taking care to include all creases and folds in the skin. Roll the child towards you to soap the back.

6. Rinse all soap off the hands, then place the left arm under the back and with the baby's head resting in the crook of the nurse's elbow, grasp the baby's left arm near the shoulder. Hold the legs with the right hand and lower the infant into the water.

The normal baby

This should be done very carefully because the skin is slippery with soap. The head must be supported while the soap is rinsed off and the baby allowed a little time in which to kick while in the water.

7. Lift the child on to the towel on the lap. Wrap up the baby and pat all over to remove excess moisture. Dry hands, arms, front, groins and legs and lightly powder. Turn the baby on to it's front, lifting the towel at the same time. Dry the back and powder, then dress the baby, tying any back fastenings. Turn on to the front and tie the front fastenings. Brush the hair. Trim the nails as necessary. The umbilical cord or stump is cleaned with mediswabs, if necessary.

N.B. When pinning a napkin the pin should be fastened in the horizontal position. In this way it is less likely to cause injury should the pin accidentally open.

Infant feeding

Wherever possible, a baby should be breast fed because human milk contains the maximum amount of nourishment required for good progress. It also contains various protective substances which ensure good health for the infant. Another great advantage is that breast fed milk is sterile and is therefore pure.

Breast-feeding mothers should be offered hospital accomodation. The nurse should ensure that the mother is made welcome and that everything possible is done for her comfort. Arrangements should be made for her to sit in a quiet place where she can relax. A comfortable chair, provided with a pillow or cushion, should be made available so that the mother can hold the baby securely.

If breast feeding cannot be maintained, small extra feeds may be given. These extra feeds may be given as follows.

Complementary feeds are given when an individual breast feed is insufficient and is followed by a small artificial feed given preferably with a spoon.

Supplementary feeds are given to replace one or more breast feeds, where the mother is unable for some reason to attend hospital for all feeds. These extra artificial feeds should be given with a spoon and should contain no sugar, to reduce the risk of refusal to take the breast.

Artificial feeding

There are many dried, milk foods prepared from cows' milk.

These foods have many advantages over liquid cows' milk. They are manufactured under hygienic conditions and are sterile in their containers. There is less risk of infection from outside sources and they are simple to store and to make up into liquid feeds as and when required.

Feeding a baby
In hospitals, prepacked feeds are used or feeds are made up in a central milk room.

All equipment used for mixing and giving the feed must be sterile.

Care must be taken that the feed is of the right temperature. Feeds may be given at room temperature or body temperature.

A jug of hot water should be placed on a trolley near the nursing chair in which to stand the feeding bottle to keep warm.

When the feed is ready, the baby should be lifted out of the cot and held comfortably in the arms whilst being fed.

As the infant takes the milk the bottle should be tilted so that the teat is constantly full of milk. If this point is not observed the child will swallow air.

The feed should be given slowly and, half-way through, the baby should be sat up for a short break to expel any wind. The remainder of the feed should then be given slowly.

When it is certain that no more wind can be expelled, the napkin is changed and the infant returned to the cot and made comfortable.

Any milk mixture not taken at the feed must be regarded as contaminated and thrown away.

The feeding bottle should be rinsed in cold water, then washed in warm soapy water, using a bottle brush, rinsed again and sterilized.

Teats should be well washed and stored in a dry, covered container labelled with the name of the baby or placed in a covered jar of sterilizing solution such as Milton 1-80, until next required. The jar containing the solution should be cleaned each day and refilled.

Teats and valves should be cleaned once a day with salt to remove the deposit left by the milk, then rinsed in plain water and returned to clean containers of Milton.

Weaning

The weaning process is one in which the milk feeds are gradually replaced by semi-solid foods in the beginning, and later by more solid foods when some of the teeth are through.

The time at which weaning is commenced depends on the age, condition and temperament of the baby. The introduction of weaning diet should begin at about 4 months. In breast-fed infants it may be even later.

New foods with new tastes should be introduced in small quantities and given with a spoon. Milk should be offered from a cup.

Plan for weaning

First week. 10 a.m. Breast or bottle feed followed by cereal. Other feeds as usual.

Second week. 2 p.m. Bone broth, vegetable puree, apple puree or rusks may be introduced.

Third week. One of the breast or bottle feeds may be discontinued to be replaced with semi-solids. A drink of milk should be offered from a cup.

Fourth week. 6 p.m. Breast or bottle feed followed by cereal, egg yolk, or soft bread and butter.

Breast or bottle feeds are gradually omitted and the feeds adjusted to coincide with normal meals. The last milk feed to be discontinued should be that taken at bedtime. The diet should contain all the food factors necessary for health (see p. 89) together with plenty of milk, fruit juices and water. Cow's milk, if used, must be boiled for children under 1 year of age. The over-use of cereals should be avoided as this can lead to excessive weight gain.

The older child

The admission of children into hospital has been discussed on page 16. If the mother has to leave for home, the child may feel bewildered and unhappy in a strange room amongst strange people. All children need love and sympathy, but in the first few hours of hospital life they are often inclined to reject any advances made by the ward staff. The successful children's nurse will fully understand this attitude and will show no impatience or resentment but will maintain a calm and friendly manner. The nurse should obtain from the relatives as much information about the child as possible with regard to favourite games or books, school friends and interests. Such information opens up a means of communication and understanding. This applies especially to the quiet child who does not cry and who gives no trouble. The barrier of silence may hide a greater sense of loss than is apparent and may lead to future ill effects. Special efforts should be made to gain the confidence of such a child. Relatives should be asked to bring a favourite toy or book which would establish a link with home.

Where possible, all children should be allowed to get up during the day and encouraged to play with each other. Some form of play activity should be provided for all children in the ward. For those confined to bed, books, pictures, jigsaw puzzles, dolls to dress and similar toys will help to distract the attention and pass the time. Play is very important to every child and must not be denied the sick child. Play leaders are now employed by most hospitals to organize play in the wards for all children, whether ambulant or confined to bed.

After the midday meal a period of rest is encouraged to ensure that the children do not become overtired.

The toilet round may prove to be an unnerving experience to a child. A chamber pot balanced on a mattress may give a child a feeling of insecurity with the result that often the bed is soiled after failure to use the pot. This may be due to the fear of overbalancing. In such cases, successful habit training may be established if the pot is placed on the floor.

Where cots or beds are soiled by excreta, no adverse comment should be made by the nurse. It is disastrous to grumble at a child in hospital for wetting the bed, whatever the age group. It must be remembered that enuresis may be temporary and may be the result of the sense of shock the child has suffered on being parted from mother and familiar surroundings. Praise given when the bed is found to be dry will have a more beneficial effect than criticism of a soiled sheet.

Safety in the children's ward

Children are naturally curious and like to explore and experiment with unknown objects. Accidents happen in an instant of time and every effort should be made to prevent them. The nurse working in a children's ward must keep a constant and alert watch on the activities of each child, especially those who are allowed out of bed. No child should be allowed out of sight of the nurse and the ward must never be left unattended.

Cot sides should be high enough to allow a small child to stand in the cot without danger of falling out. The sides should be locked into position to prevent them dropping and at no time should they be left down. Restrainers should not be used unless absolutely necessary, but where essential they should be made to fasten at the back so that the child cannot untie them. They must not be attached to the cot sides as this could result in injury to the child.

Babies under 1 year old should not have a soft pillow because of the danger of suffocation. Plastic bibs or plastic bags may also cause suffocation.

Windows should be closed at the bottom or barred, to prevent children from falling or climbing through.

Heavy doors should be fastened so that fingers are not crushed as they close.

Children should not be allowed in the bathroom without supervision. The bathroom door should be kept closed when not in use. Hot-water taps should be operated by a removable key which should be hung out of reach. Bathroom doors should not have bolts or locks on the insides.

All cupboards should be locked. No medicines or lotions of any kind should be left in the ward or annexes.

All radiators should be protected with a guard.

Electric points should be fixed on the wall out of reach, and should be covered, as a further precaution.

Toys small enough to put into the mouth should not be given to a child. Larger toys with detachable parts which might be swallowed should also be prohibited.

Jugs or bowls of hot liquids must not be left within reach of any child.

Care should be taken when meal trolleys are in the ward.

Hot drinks should not be given to a child until cool enough to drink or hold without danger of scalding.

Any accidents must be reported immediately, however slight. The ward sister will notify the parents as soon as possible.

26
First aid treatment in emergencies

The objects of first aid are to give immediate and temporary care in cases of accident or sudden illness, to prevent further injury, to assist recovery and to arrange for the patient to receive skilled help as soon as possible, either from a doctor or in hospital. The speed with which the patient is placed under medical care is of the greatest importance to recovery and may be the means of saving life.

General rules of first aid

These rules are given as a guide to the care of a casualty. Varying circumstances may require the application of some or all of them. The first aider must be prepared to adapt the treatment to the conditions under which the accident or illness occurs and to the immediate needs of the patient.

1. Send for a doctor, the police or an ambulance.
2. Conditions endangering life must be dealt with first. These are failure in breathing, haemorrhage and severe shock, in that order. If breathing has stopped, artifical respiration must be started without delay and continued until medical aid is available. Every second counts in saving the life of the casualty.
3. Reassure the casualty if conscious. This is important because injured people or those overtaken by sudden illness are usually very frightened. Reassurance given in a quiet and confident manner will often help in reducing the degree of shock.
4. Fresh air is essential. Onlookers should be prevented from crowding round and should be tactfully requested to refrain from passing comments on the apparent condition of the casualty.
5. Loosen tight clothing but do not remove clothing unnecessarily. The patient should be disturbed as little as possible, unless there is danger from other sources, such as

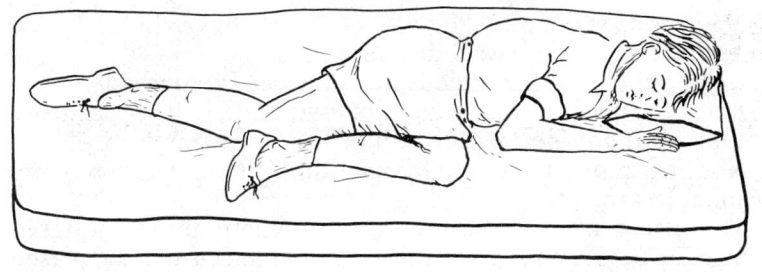

Fig. 26.1 Position for unconscious patient.

falling walls or masonry, escaping gas, electric current or passing traffic.

6. Unless injuries are too severe, an unconscious patient should be turned on the side to prevent the tongue from falling backwards over the larynx (p. 50 and Fig. 26.1).

Causes of unconsciousness

1. Apoplexy is the result of cerebral haemorrhage, cerebral thrombosis or cerebral embolism (see p. 161).
2. Asphyxia from drowning, choking, strangulation or suffocation by poisonous gases or smoke.
3. Diabetic or insulin coma (see p. 214).
4. Epilepsy (see p. 165).
5. Excessive heat.
6. Fainting.
7. Haemorrhage.
8. Head injury with concussion or compression of the brain.
9. Infantile convulsions.
10. Poisoning by chemicals.
11. Shock.

Shock

The word shock is a loose term used to describe the state in which the patient, for whatever reason, has peripheral circulatory collapse. This results in a cold, clammy skin and pallor. The patient usually feels faint (or may be unconscious) has a rapid, feeble pulse, low blood pressure and shallow respirations. He may vomit.

Treatment of shock

Place the casualty flat with the feet raised.

If the patient is unconscious, turn the head to one side.

Keep the patient warm but not overheated. If the casualty becomes too hot, body fluids will be lost in perspiration.

Nothing must be given by mouth if the patient requires hospital treatment.

The effect of shock causes acute anxiety to the sufferer. Much can be done to lessen this by reassurance from the person caring for him.

The casualty should be removed to hospital as soon as possible.

First aid treatments

Apoplexy

The patient should be made comfortable, placed on his side to maintain a clear airway, and removed to hospital as soon as possible.

Asphyxia

Asphyxia is a dangerous condition in which the lungs are deprived of oxygen and the vital organs, i.e. the heart and the brain, are affected. Unless the supply of oxygen is rapidly restored by artificial respiration, death will occur.

Drowning

Using a handkerchief over a finger, clear the mouth of any mud or weed. Turn the casualty face downwards and proceed with artificial respiration without delay and continue until breathing starts again. If help can be obtained, the wet clothing should be gradually removed and the patient covered with any dry coverings available.

Choking

To remove a foreign body lodged in the throat, bend the casualty's head forward and strike the back hard beneath the shoulder blades. A small child can be held upside down whilst doing this. If this method fails, induce vomiting by irritating the back of the throat with a finger.

Strangulation

Cut and remove the band constricting the throat and apply artificial respiration. On recovery from strangulation the tissues of the throat may be swollen. If conscious, give sips of cold water. Send for medical aid.

Hanging

Help will be needed to support the weight of the body before cutting it down. Artificial respiration must be tried until the arrival of the police or a doctor.

Suffocation by gas

Before entering a room full of gas, take a deep breath and hold it. Open doors and windows in the room. If necessary break the window with the heel of a shoe. Pull the casualty out into the air and apply artificial respiration. Send for a doctor or an ambulance.

Suffocation by smoke

The rescuer should tie a wet cloth round the mouth and nose and enter the room keeping the head as near to the ground as possible. Pull the casualty out into the fresh air and apply artificial respiration if breathing has ceased.

Electric shock

Switch off the current. If this is not possible, pull out the plug or protect a hand with thick newspaper and break the cable. *Cables must not be cut with scissors or knives.* Water, dampness or metal will conduct the electric current to the rescuer unless he is well protected. Before touching the casualty, the hands must be covered with thick newspaper, woollen material or rubber and the feet placed on material of the same kind or on a wooden board. A walking-stick with no metal attachments may be used to drag the casualty away from the live wire. If breathing has stopped, apply artificial respiration, send for a doctor or an ambulance and treat the patient for shock.

Heat exhaustion and heat stroke

Place the patient in a cool place, Loosen the clothing and apply a cold compress to the head. If conscious, give salted water to drink (a ¼ teaspoonful of salt to a glass of water). The patient should be put to bed as soon as possible and tepid sponged (see p. 25). The body temperature must not be allowed to fall too suddenly.

Fainting

If the patient feels faint, have her sitting or lying down with the head lower than the knees. If unconscious, place the patient flat on the floor in a current of fresh air and loosen any tight clothing. On recovery, sips of water may be given.

Haemorrhage (see also p. 65)

Arterial and venous haemorrhage may endanger life and must be treated without delay. Pressure may be applied directly over the wound using the fingers or a pad and bandage. If this fails to stop the bleeding, pressure must be applied over the nearest pressure point between the site of the injury and the heart. A pressure point is where an artery crosses a bone and can be pressed against it to stop the flow of blood from below that point.

General rules for the arrest of haemorrhage
 1. Send for a doctor or an ambulance.
 2. Place the casualty flat, unless there is bleeding from the head or neck, in which case the head should be slightly raised. If there is no fracture, raise and support the injured limb to lessen the flow of blood to the part.
 3. Do not remove any blood clots because they assist in checking the haemorrhage.
 4. Apply direct or indirect pressure as required.
 5. Apply a pad and bandage and immobilize the injured part, using a splint if necessary.

Pressure points
Carotid pressure point (Fig. 26.2) to control bleeding from the head and neck. Place the thumb in the hollow between the lower part of the larynx and the sterno-mastoid muscle and exert firm pressure upwards and backwards towards the vertebrae.
 Subclavian pressure point (Fig. 26.3) for haemorrhage from the upper arm and shoulder. Press both thumbs into the hollow

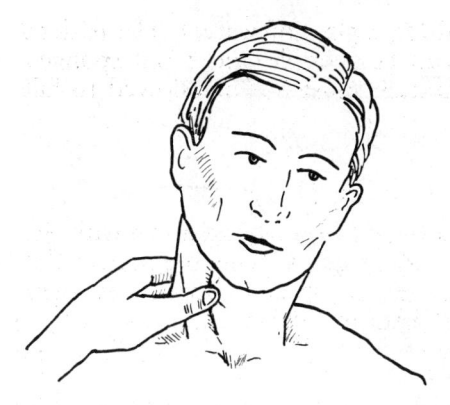

Fig. 26.2 Carotid pressure point.

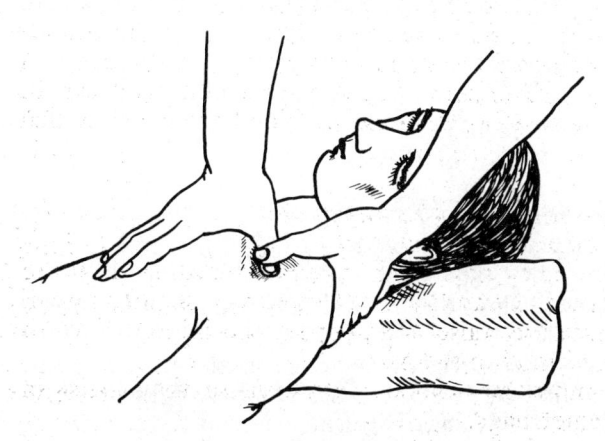

Fig. 26.3 Subclavian pressure point.

above the clavicle and compress the artery against the first rib. Turn the patient's head toward the injured side.

Brachial pressure point (Fig. 26.4) to control bleeding from the arm. Pass the hand under the arm and compress the brachial artery against the humerus in an upward and backward direction.

Femoral pressure point (Fig. 26.5). The femoral artery passes through the groin and down the inside of the thigh. To stop haemorrhage from the leg, bend the casualty's knee, grip the thigh in the centre of the groin with both hands compressing

238 Practical nursing

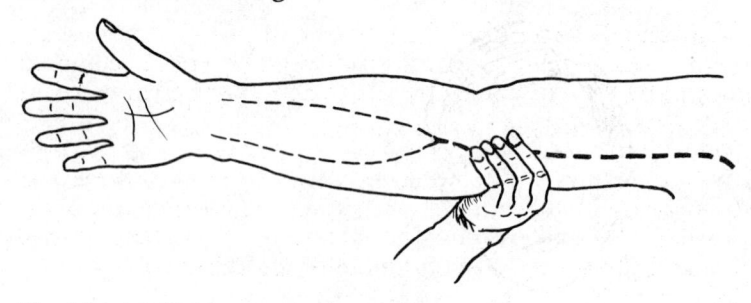

Fig. 26.4 Brachial-artery pressure point.

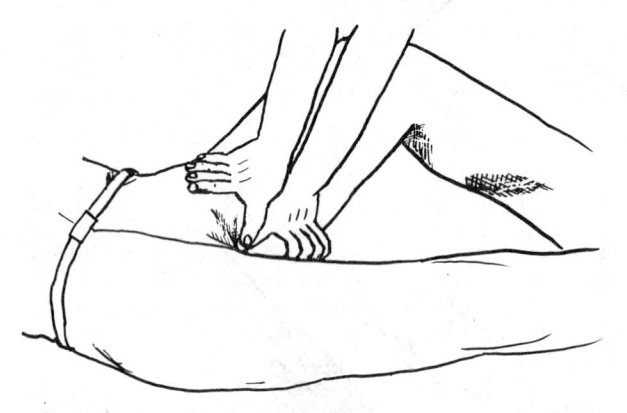

Fig. 26.5 Femoral-artery pressure point.

the femoral artery against the pelvic bone. The thumbs should be placed one over the other for greater pressure.

A *tourniquet* is a constrictive bandage used where bleeding cannot be controlled by other means, or where pressure must be maintained for any length of time. A tourniquet can be made with a belt, braces or any soft material placed round the limb above the bleeding part and over the clothing. A loose knot is tied and a stick, pen or pencil inserted into the knot and twisted until the bleeding is checked. Any type of tourniquet must be released every fifteen minutes to allow the blood to circulate or injury to other vessels and nerves may result. If haemorrhage persists, the tourniquet can be tightened again. When a patient is removed to hospital with a tourniquet in place, a note must be sent with the patient stating the position and the time it was last released. A large T marked on the forehead with lipstick or a pen will attract the attention of ambulance or hospital staffs. A tourniquet must *not* be used unless absolutely necessary.

Venous haemorrhage, as from a ruptured varicosed vein, may be controlled by raising the limb and applying a firm pad and bandage over the part.

Head injuries should be regarded as serious, even though unconsciousness is only momentary. The patient should be strongly advised to keep quiet and to consult a doctor as soon as possible. If unconsciousness intervenes, treat for shock, apply a dressing to any wounds and send for a doctor.

Infantile convulsions

Apply the general rules for unconsciousness and send for a doctor. Tepid sponge the child if the temperature is elevated. When the convulsion has passed, put the child in a quiet place to sleep.

Poisons

Keep any container or sample or the poison, also any vomited material, and send to the hospital with the casualty.

If conscious and the lips and mouth are burnt, give water or milk to drink. Remove urgently to hospital.

If unconscious, place in the recovery position.

If breathing has ceased, begin resuscitation. Remove urgently to hospital.

Do not induce vomiting in either group of patients. Do not waste time looking for antidotes.

Artificial respiration

Aim

The aim is to maintain adequate oxygenation and circulation of the blood. Speed is essential; if the brain is deprived of oxygen for more than four minutes, permanent damage will result.

Emergency resuscitation (Fig. 26.6)

Mouth to mouth method

This is the most effective method. Contra-indications may be:
1. severe facial injury;
2. active vomiting;
3. casualty trapped face down.

240 *Practical nursing*

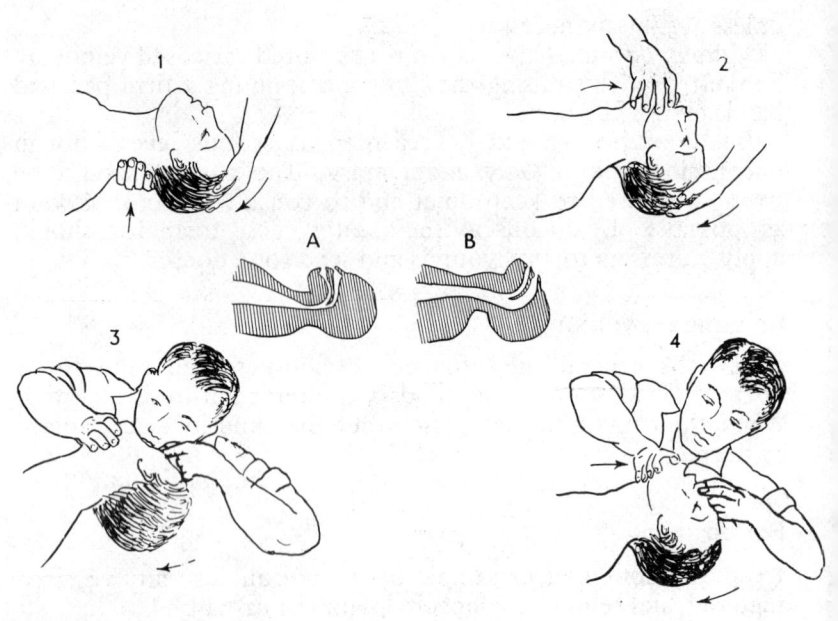

Fig. 26.6 Artificial respiration, mouth to mouth.

Place the casualty on his back and work from the side. Clear the mouth and nose of any debris. Tilt the head backwards by pressing the top of the head downwards with one hand and pushing the jaw upwards with the other. Keeping the jaw upwards with one hand, pinch the nostrils with the other.

Take a deep breath and seal the lips round the casualty's mouth and blow with the mouth wide open while obstructing the casualty's nostrils with the cheek. It may be necessary to pinch the nostrils together.

Watch for the chest to rise, then lift your head to let the air escape from the lungs.

The first ten inflations should be given quickly, after which they should be given at ten to twelve times a minute. If beginning to feel dizzy, the rescuer should proceed at a slower rate.

For an infant or young child the nose and mouth should be covered with the lips and the rate increased to twenty times a minute. The neck of an infant or young child should be less acutely extended than in an adult otherwise obstruction will result.

First aid treatment in emergencies 241

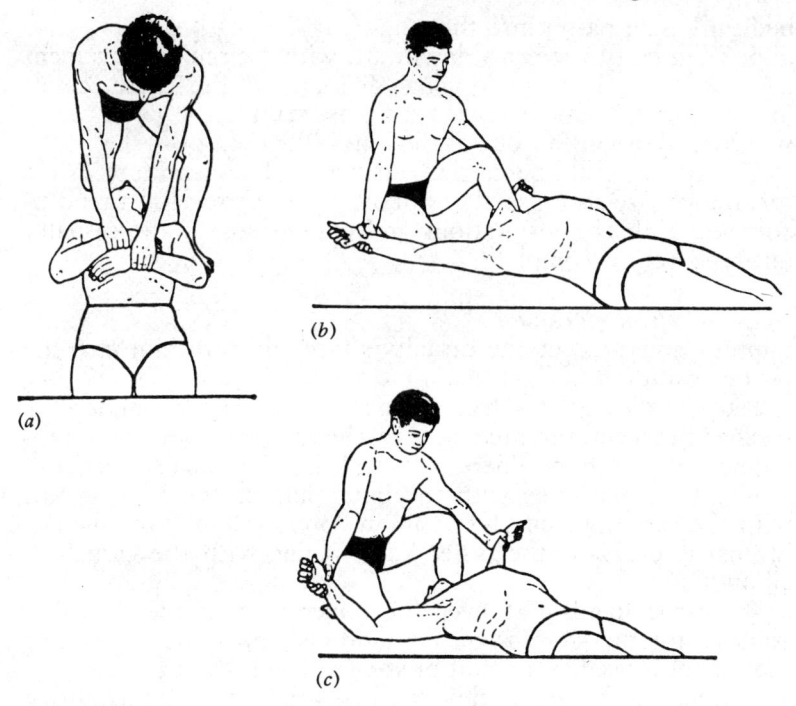

Fig. 26.7 Sylvester's method of artificial respiration. (From *Artificial Respiration Handbook*. Royal Life Saving Society, London.)

Sylvester's method (Fig. 26.7)
The casualty is placed on the back with a thick pad made of rolled-up coats or blankets placed underneath the shoulder blades. The neck should be well extended with the head thrown back and barely touching the ground.

The rescuer kneels on the right knee in line with the right side of the casualty's head with the left foot placed at the level of the casualty's left shoulder. Proceed as follows.

1. Grasp the patient's wrists and cross them just below the lower end of the sternum.
2. Keeping the arms straight, rock gently forward to exert an even pressure on the chest (count 'one') (Fig. 26.7a).
3. Rock backwards lifting the casualty's arms outwards and upwards in a circular movement until they extend above the head (counting 'two'). The arms must be kept clear of the ground and the upward movement stopped when resistance is felt. This enlarges the cavity of the chest and inspiration may

be heard as air passes into the lungs (Fig. 26.7b).

4. Then carry the arms downward with a circular movement and place them in the original position on the chest (count 'one'). This movement lowers the ribs, making the chest cavity smaller and driving air out of the lungs (Fig. 26.7c).

The cycle should be carried out twelve times a minute. When breathing is re-established the movements should be timed to coincide with the inspirations and expirations of the casualty until recovery is complete.

Holger-Nielson method

Support and protect the casualty's face and turn him into the prone position.

Place the casualty's hands, one over the other, under the forehead to keep the face clear of the ground. Give three sharp slaps between the shoulder-blades to bring the tongue forward.

Kneel on one knee with the inner side of the knee in line with the casualty's cheek and about 25 cm (10 in) from the top of his head. Place the other knee in line with the casualty's elbow.

Place the hands flat over the lower part of the shoulder-blades with the thumbs on each side of the spine. A rocking movement is used to a count of six. Force must not be used.

1. Keeping the arms straight, rock gently forward counting 'one-two' (two seconds). This causes expiration.

2. Rock back, counting 'three' (one second), sliding the hands past the casualty's shoulders to grip the arms near the elbows. Do not raise the chest from the ground.

3. Raise and pull on the arms counting 'four-five' (two seconds). This movement causes inspiration.

4. Counting 'six' (one second), lower the casualty's arms to the ground and replace the hands in the original position over the shoulder-blades.

The complete procedure takes six seconds and must be repeated ten times a minute.

Where artificial respiration must be continued for some hours, the operator may change from one knee to the other, but the rhythm of the movements must not change or stop for even a second. A second operator may relieve the first by kneeling on the other side of the casualty and placing the hands over those of the first operator on the casualty's shoulder-blade, continuing the movements with the same rhythm and without a break.

For children the movements are the same, but pressure on

the back is applied with the finger-tips only.

For children under 5 years old, the forehead should be supported on a folded coat or cloth to keep the face clear of the ground and the arms placed at the sides. The shoulders should be held by the operator with the fingers underneath and the thumbs on the back of the shoulder. Press the thumbs on the back, counting 'one-two', then lift the shoulders slightly counting 'three-four' at a rate of fifteen times per minute. The child may be placed on a table with the operator standing at the head.

External cardiac compression
If the heart is not beating, put the casualty on his back on a firm surface. Strike the left side of chest with the edge of your hand. If the heart does not start beating, start external cardiac compression immediately.
Method
Kneel at one side of the casualty. Place the heel of one hand on the lower half of the sternum, keeping the palm and fingers off the chest. Place the heel of the other hand on top of the first hand. Keeping your arms straight, rock forward and press on the lower half of sternum.

Release pressure and allow sternum to spring back.

Repeat pressure sixty times per minute for an adult.

In children, the pressure of one hand is sufficient and the rate should be about eighty times per minute.

In infants **light** pressure with two fingers is all that is required and the rate should be about one hundred times per minute.
Indications of effective treatment
   1. Improvement of casualty's colour.
   2. Constriction of previously dilated pupils.
   3. Palpable carotid pulse.
N.B. Both cardiac and respiratory resuscitation should be carried out simultaneously.

Four cardiac compressions to one lung inflation is the usual rate.

Other emergencies

Bee and wasp stings

Remove the sting with forceps or tweezers. For a bee sting, apply a solution of bicarbonate of soda, blue bag or methylated spirits. A wasp sting should be treated with a weak solution of vinegar or lemon juice. If the tongue or mouth are stung, a mouth wash made with 1 teaspoonful of bicarbonate of soda to a glass of water or ice to suck may be given. Take the patient to a doctor. If the patient has breathing difficulties, place in the recovery position.

Burns

If the clothing is in flames, the rescuer should approach the casualty holding a thick blanket, rug or coat in front of himself to give protection, then wrap it round the victim, lay him flat, and smother the flames.

Emergency treatment of burns
1. Remove clothing soaked in boiling fluids. Do not remove dry burnt clothing.
2. To reduce the effects of heat, the area should be placed below slowly running water for at least ten minutes. If this is not possible, pour cold water from a jug over the area. It is important to continue for at least ten minutes to stop the effects of heat on the tissues.
3. Remove anything constrictive, e.g. watch, ring, shoes, before swelling begins.
4. Do not prick blisters.
5. Cover the area with clean dressing or linen.
6. If serious, arrange for immediate removal to hospital.
7. Any patient requiring hospital treatment should not be given anything by mouth.

Burns from corrosives
Quickly remove any clothing on which the corrosive has spilled and flood the burned area gently with water to remove as much as possible of the chemical.

Take care not to contaminate yourself. Remove to hospital.

Scalds of the mouth or throat

These occur when a child drinks from the spout of a boiling kettle or teapot. Send for an ambulance immediately. Keep the child as warm and as quiet as possible. Give ice to suck or very cold water to drink, if conscious. Maintain a clear airway.

Dog bites

Squeeze the blood toward the punctured wound and wash well. Cover with a clean dressing and take the patient to a doctor.

First aid treatment in emergencies

The condition and behaviour of the dog should be noted, if possible, and reported. If rabies is suspected, the patient will have to be immunized against the disease.

Foreign bodies

In the eye
Grit or dust which can be seen in the eye may be removed with the corner of a clean handkerchief, moistened in water. A drop of castor oil will relieve any soreness. If the foreign body appears to be sticking to the eye, no attempt must be made to remove the foreign body by other means. Cover the affected eye and take the casualty to hospital.

In the nose
Beads, buttons or marbles may be discharged if the patient is made to sneeze with a little pepper or snuff. If this is not successful medical help must be sought. No attempt must be made to remove the foreign body by other means.

In the ear
An insect in the ear may be floated out with a little olive oil or salad oil poured into the ear. Any other foreign body in the ear *must be left severely alone and no attempt made to remove it*. The patient must consult a doctor.

In the stomach
Pins, needles, buttons, screws, etc., may be swallowed. Seek medical advice. Do **not** give anything by mouth.

Bandaging

Netelast (Fig. 26.8)
Netelast is the modern type of bandage composed of cotton and elastic in the form of a wide-mesh tubular net. It is made in different sizes according to the area of the body to be bandaged. The elastic fibres hold the dressing in place and can be turned back for renewal of the dressing without undue disturbance of the patient.

Tubegauz (Fig. 26.9)
Tubegauz is another method of bandaging now used in many hospitals. It is manufactured in seamless rolls of tubular gauze

(a)

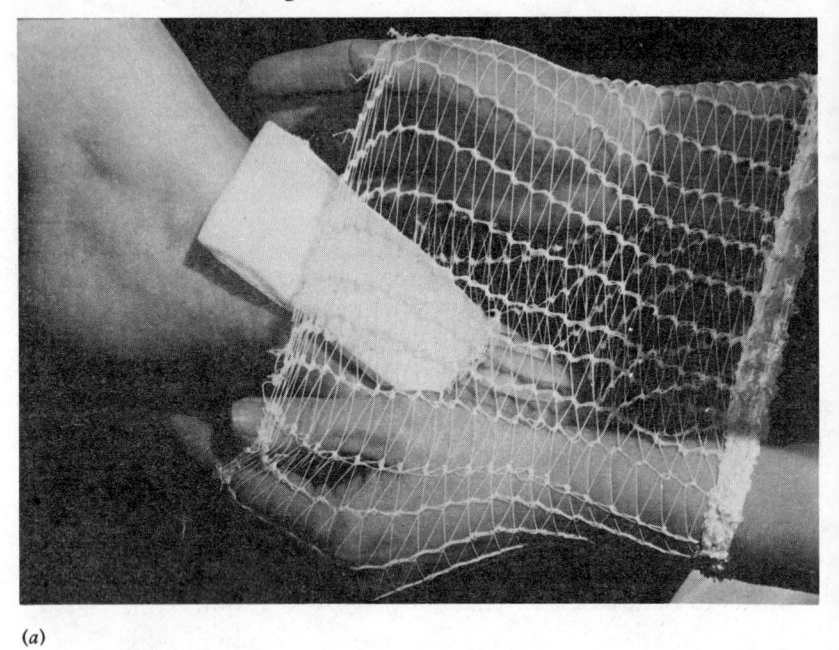

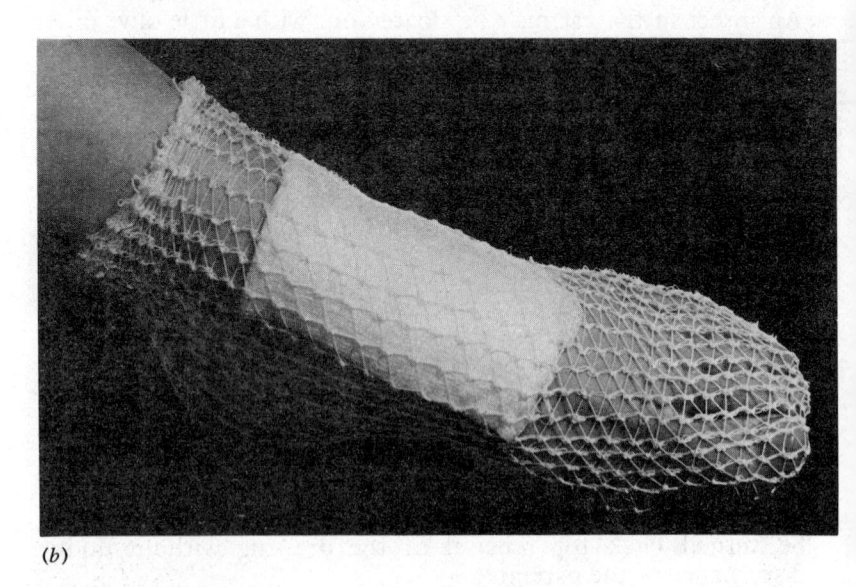

(b)

Fig. 26.8 Illustrations to show various uses of Netelast.

First aid treatment in emergencies

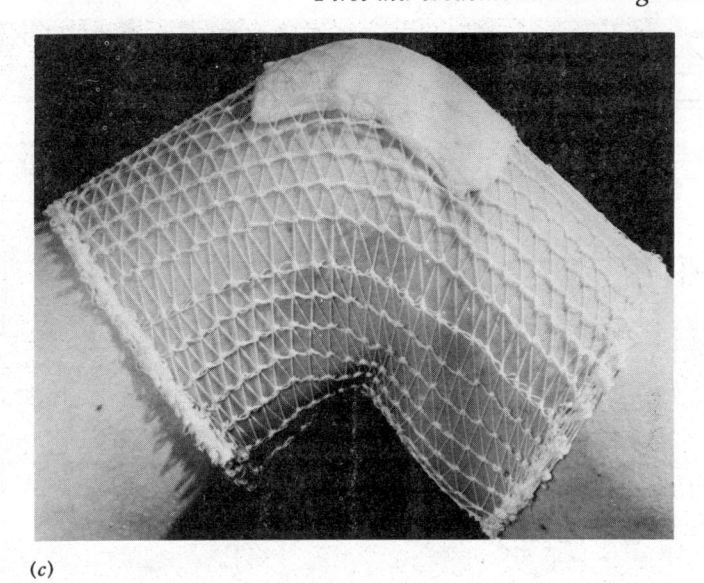

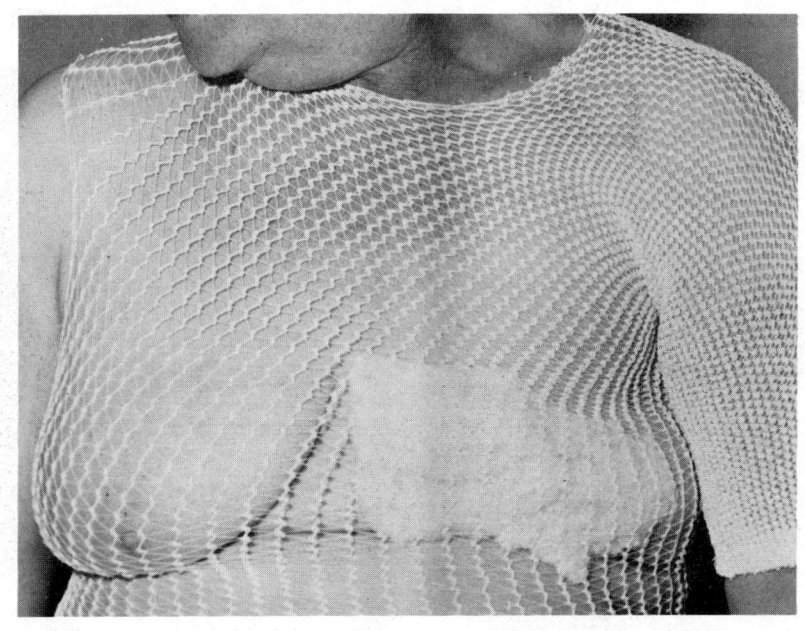

(c)

(d)

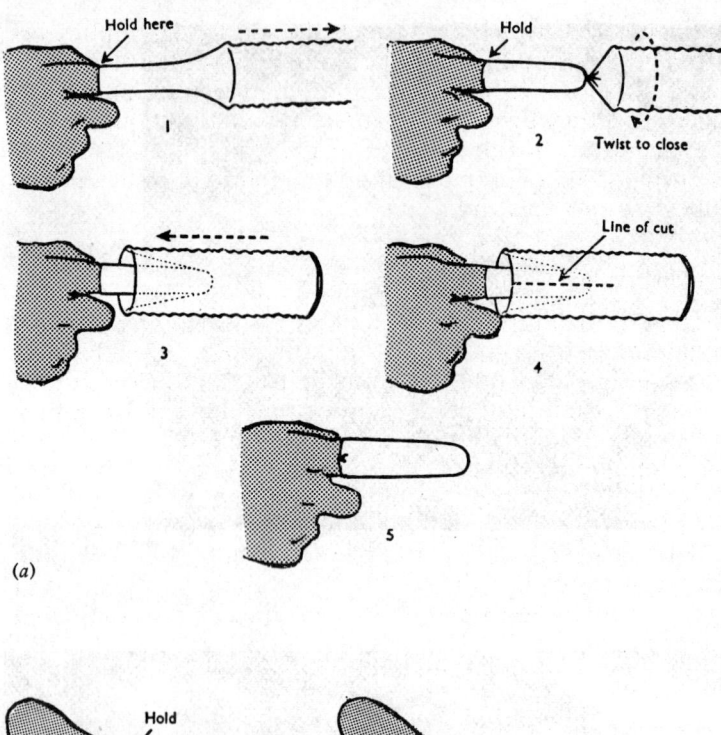

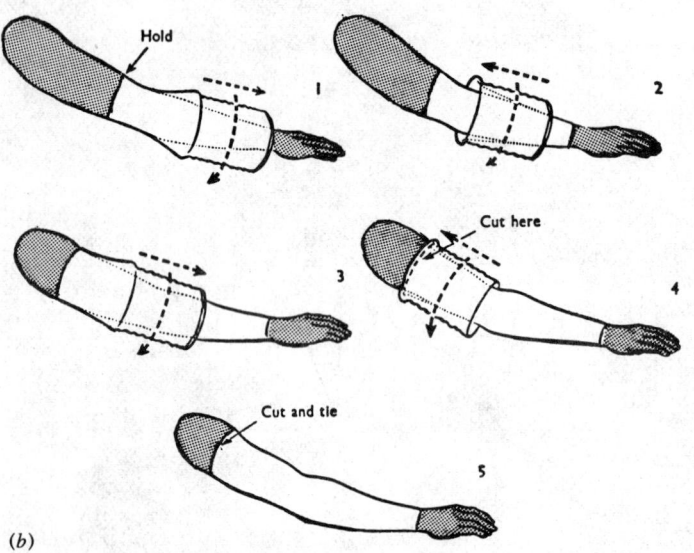

Fig. 26.9 Tubegauz. (Scholl Manufacturing Co. Ltd.)

of various widths, which are stretched over special applicators of different sizes to fit any part of the body. For general purposes, Tubegauz, about twice the length of the part to be bandaged, is gathered on to the applicator of the requisite size and applied over the dressing. The completed bandage may be fastened with a small piece of adhesive plaster or by cutting the Tubegauz into tails and tying.

Triangular bandages and slings

The triangular bandage may be used as a sling to give support to an injured arm or hand, to keep dressings in place over large areas, e.g. the chest or groin or to completely cover a hand, foot or the scalp. In first aid, triangular bandages may be used to secure splints in position.

To tie the ends of a bandage, a flat reef knot must be used. This is made by taking an end of the bandage or sling in each hand. Cross the end in the right hand over and under the end in the left hand. Then cross the end in the left hand over and under that in the right hand. (Right over and under the left and left over and under the right.) Tuck the ends of the completed knot out of sight.

Broad sling for the arm (Fig. 26.10)
Place the point of the bandage under the elbow on the injured side. Flex the elbow into a comfortable position. Pass the end

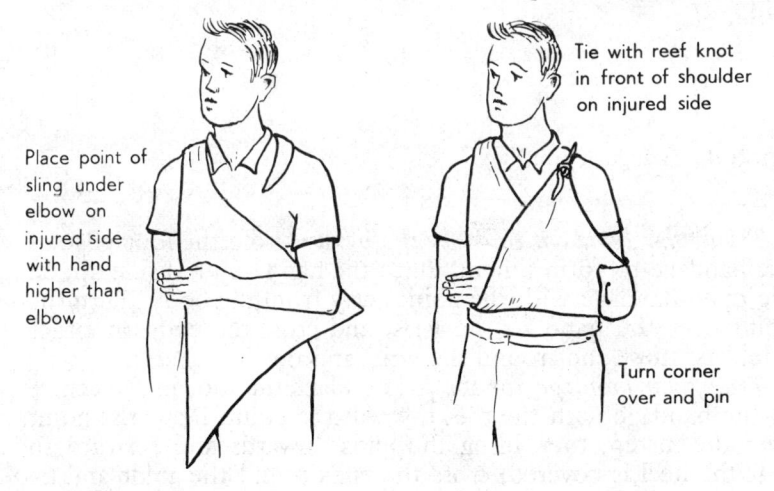

Fig. 26.10 Arm sling.

of the bandage, nearest the body round the back of the neck to the front of the shoulder on the injured side. Carry the other end up to meet the first end and tie a reef knot in the hollow above the clavicle. Tuck the bandage in behind the elbow, bring the point forward and fasten with a safety pin.

Trianuglar sling (Fig. 26.11)
Place the arm across the chest with the fingers touching the opposite clavicle. Lay the open bandage across the front of the chest and over the arm, with the point well beyond the elbow. Tuck the lower part of the bandage under the hand and arm and bring the end upwards across the back to meet the other end. Tie in the hollow above the clavicle on the uninjured side.

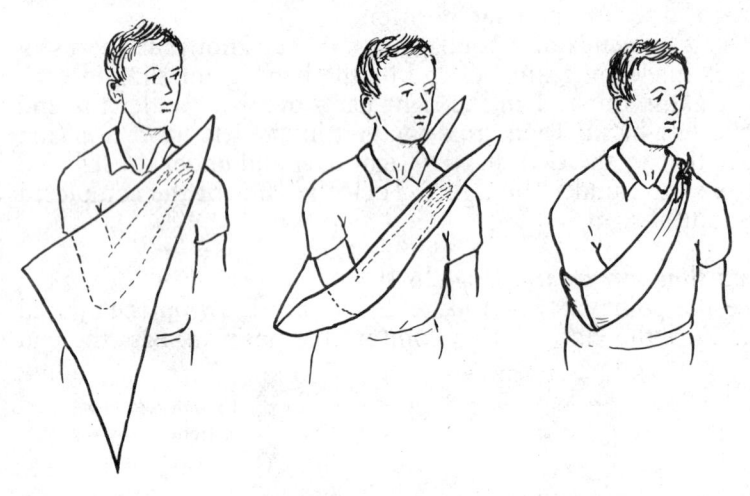

Fig. 26.11 Triangular arm sling.

Triangular bandage to cover the hand Fold the long edge of the bandage to form a hem. Place the hand, injured side up, on the open bandage with the point away from the body. Turn the point over the hand to the wrist and cross the ends on either side. Pass these ends round the wrist and tie.

Triangular bandage for the foot Place the foot in the centre of the bandage with the toes towards the point. Draw the point over the instep, then bring the ends upwards and forward so that the heel is covered, cross the ends round the ankle and tie in front.

First aid treatment in emergencies 251

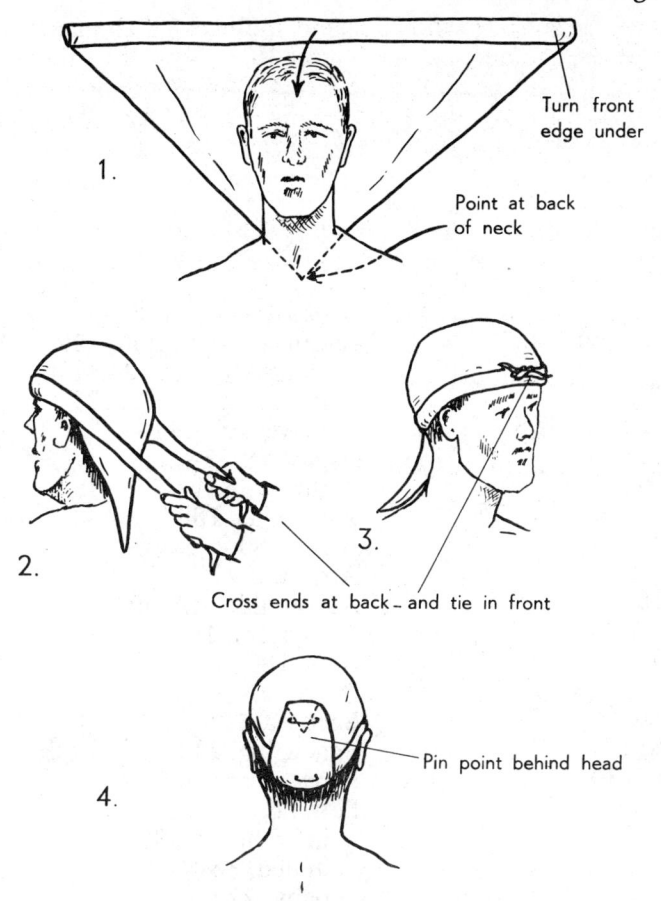

Fig. 26.12 Triangular head bandage.

Triangular bandage for the head (Fig. 26.12) Place the long side of the bandage over the forehead, cross the ends at the back and tie in front. Bring the point up to the back of the head and fasten near the top of the scalp. This bandage can be adapted to cover the knee, elbow or shoulder.

Index

Abscess, 74
Acetabulum, 186
Acne, 46
Acromegaly, 115
Addison's disease, 118
Administration of
 medicines, 119
Admission of patients, 15
Adrenal glands, 118
Air hunger, 27
Amylase, 101
Analgesics, 124
Anaemia, 73
Anaesthetics, 124
Angina pectoris, 68
Antibiotics, 124
Antibodies, 130
Anticoagulants, 125
Antidotes, 125
Anus, 93
Aorta, 59
Aperients, 125
Apoplexy, 234
Appendicitis, 98
Appendix, 98
Approach to the patient, 3
Aqueous humour, 169
Arachnoid membrane, 159
Arteries, 61
Arterio-sclerosis, 68
Arthritis, 190
Artificial feeding, 109
 infants, 227
 gastrostomy, 110

 naso-gastric, 108
Artificial respiration, 239
 Holgar Neilson, 242
 mouth to mouth, 239
 Sylvester's 241
Asphyxia, 234
Asthma, 56
Astragalus, 188
Atlas, 180
Atrium, 59
Autonomic nervous
 system, 160
Axis, 180

Bacteria, 126
Bandaging, 245
Barrier nursing, 129
Bathing,
 in bathroom, 37
 in bed, 38
 baby, 225
B.C.G., 217
Bedding, 9
Bedmaking, 10
Beds, special, 12
Bedsores, 42
Behaviour, 20
Beriberi, 90
Biceps, 153
Bile, 99
Bladder, gall, 100
 urinary, 78
Blepharitis, 170
Blood, 71

Index 253

grouping, 72
pressure, 69
transfusion, 72
Boils, 46
Bones, 122
Brain, 157
  diseases of, 161
  injury to, 197
Bronchi, 51
Bronchiectasis, 56
Bronchitis, 53
Broncho-pneumonia, 54
Burns, first aid in, 244
  hospital treatment, 210

Caecostomy, 34
Caecum, 98
Calories, 104
Capillaries, 62
Carbohydrates, 89
Carbon-dioxide, 50
Carcinoma, 215
Carpal bones, 185
Carriers, 128
Cartilage, 152
  articular, 189
  intervertebral, 179
  thyroid, 50
  tracheal, 51
Cataract, 170
Catheterization, 83
Cells, 150
  blood, 71
  lymph, 112
Centigrade thermometer, 21
Cerebellum, 158
Cerebrospinal fluid, 159
Cerebrum, 158
Chancre, 218
Cheyne Stoke's
  breathing, 27
Chicken-pox, 132
Children in hospital, 224
  admission of, 16

Choking, 234
Cholecystitis, 107
Choroid, 168
Circulation of blood, 59
Cleanliness,
  annexes, 7
  kitchen, 7
  patient, 38
  personal, 2
Clavicle, 186
  fracture of, 198
Clinical thermometer, 20
Clips,
  Kifa, 149
  Michel, 148
Coccyx, 179
Cochlea, 176
Cold compress, 76
Colic, 156
Colles' fracture, 198
Colostomy, 34
Coma, diabetic, 214
  insulin, 214
Complementary
  feeding, 227
Conjunctiva, 168
Conjunctivitis, 170
Connective tissue, 153
Convulsions, 239
Cornea, 168
Corns, 46
Coronary arteries, 61
Coronary thrombosis, 68
Coryza, 53
Cough, 20
Cranial nerves, 159
Cranium, 181
Cretinism, 116
Cries of children, 224
Cross infection, 142
CSSD, 137
Cyanosis, 18
Cystitis, 87

Dangerous drugs, 119
  classification of, 124
  storage and
    administration of, 119
Dermatitis, 46
Dermis, 36
Diabetes mellitus, 211
Diastole, 70
Diets, 104
Digestive system, 93
  disorders of, 106
Digestive process, 101
Diphtheria, 134
Discharge of patients, 17
Disinfection, 136
Diuretics, 125
Dog bite, 244
Dressings, 143
Droplet infection, 127
Drops, eye, 172
Drowning, 234
Drugs,
  by inhalation, 118
  by injection, 123
  by inunction, 119
  by mouth, 120
  per rectum, 30
Duodenum, 97
Dura mater, 159
Dyspepsia, 106
Dysuria, 30

Ear, 174
  foreign body in, 245
Eczema, 46
Elbow, 185
Electric shock, 235
Embolism, 69
Emetics, 125
Emphysema, 54
Emphyema, 54
Endocarditis, 67
Endocardium, 61
Endocrine glands, 115

Enemata, 30
  special, 31
Enteritis, 108
Enuresis, 80
Enzymes, 101
Epidemic, 131
Epidermis, 36
Epididymis, 202
Epiglottis, 50
Epilepsy, 165
Epiphysis, 152
Epistaxis, 65
Epithelium, 150
Erysipelas, 47
Erythema, 45
Ethmoid bone, 183
Etiquette, 3
Eustachian tubes, 96, 115
Evaporating compress, 76
Expectorants, 125
Eye, 168
  artificial, 171
  drops, 172
  foreign body in, 245
  hot bathing of, 171
  irrigation, 172

Face, bones of, 183
Faeces, 19
Fainting, 236
Fallopian tubes, 204
Feeding, 102
  artificial, 109
  helpless patients, 102
  infant, 227
Feet, bones of, 188
  care of, 2
Femur, 186
Fibrositis, 154
Fibula, 188
Fire prevention, 57
First aid, 232
Flat foot, 189
Flatus tube, 32

Index

Fluid balance, 82
Fomites, 127
Fontanelles, 132
Food,
   classes of, 89
   serving of, 102
Foramen magnum, 183
Foreign bodies, 245
Fractures, 193
Fracture bed, 12
Frequency of
   micturition, 79

Gall bladder, 100
Gas poisoning, 235
Gastric juice, 101
Gastro-enteritis, 129
Geriatric nursing, 206
German measles, 132
Gigantism, 115
Glands,
   adrenal, 118
   lymph, 112
   mammary, 204
   parathyroid, 117
   pituitary, 115
   prostate, 203
   salivary, 95
   sex, 115
   sweat, 36
   thymus, 118
   thyroid, 116
Gonorrhoea, 219
Gout, 191
Grave's disease, 117
Gynaecological procedures, 204

Haemoglobin, 71
Haematemesis, 65
Haematoma, 66
Haematuria, 66
Haemoptysis, 65

Haemorrhage, 65, 236
Hair, care of, 40
Hands, bones of, 185
   care of, 2
Hanging, 285
Heaf test, 217
Heat stroke, 235
Heart, 59
   diseases of, 67
Hemiplegia, 161
Herpes, 39
Herpes zoster, 47, 166
Hiccough, 21
Hodgkin's disease, 114
Humerus, 186
Hydrochloric acid, 101
Hygiene,
   communal, 128, 217
   personal, 2
Hyoid bone, 183
Hyperglycaemia, 214
Hyperpyrexia, 23
Hypnotics, 125
Hypoglycaemia, 214
Hypostatic pneumonia, 54

Ileum, 98
Ilium, 186
Incus, 174
Immunization, 129
Impetigo, 47
Incontinence, 79
Incubation, 131
Infant,
   bathing, 225
   feeding, 227
   weaning, 228
Inflammation, 75
Inhalations, 56
Infection,
   prevention of, 128
   sources of, 127
   spread of, 127
Infectious diseases, 132

Infusions,
 intravenous, 124
Injections,
 hypodermic, 123
 intramuscular, 121
 intravenous, 123
Innominate bones, 186
Instruments, 141, 148
Insulin, 212
Intervertebral, disc, 179
Inunctions, 119
Iodine, 90
Iris, 168
Iron, in blood, 71
 in food, 90
Ischium, 186
Islets of Langerhans, 99
Isolation, 129

Jaundice, 108
Jejenum, 98

Kaolin poultice, 75
Kidneys, 77
Kitchen, 7
Knee, 186
Koplik's spots, 132

Lacrimal, bones, 183
 ducts, 168
 glands, 168
Laryngitis, 53
Larynx, 50
Last offices, 220
Lens, 168
Leucocytes, 71
Leukaemia, 74
Lipase, 101
Liver, 99
Lumbago, 156
Lumbar puncture, 163
Lungs, 51
Lymph, 112
Lymphatic system, 112

Macule, 45
Malar bone, 183
Malleolus, 188
Mallet, 174
Mammary glands, 204
Mantoux test, 217
Marrow, 71, 177
Maxillary bones, 183
Meals, serving of, 102
Measles, 132
Medicine, administration
 of, 119
Medulla oblongata, 159
Melaena, 66
Membranes, 150
Meninges, 159
Mental welfare,
 chronic sick, 208
 elderly, 206
 pre-operative, 138
Metabolism, 89
Metacarpal bones, 185
Metatarsal bones, 188
Micturition, 79
Milk, 91
 classes of, 92
Mineral salts, 90
Misuse of Drugs Act, 119
Mitral stenosis, 67
Monoplegia, 161
Mouth, 83
 care of, 39
Multiple sclerosis, 165
Mumps, 133
Muscular system, 153
 disorders of, 155
Myocarditis, 67
Myocardium, 60
Myxoedema, 117

Nails, care of, 2
Narcotics, 125
Nasal bones, 183
Naso-pharynx, 51

Nausea, 19
Neoplasms, 215
Nephritis, 86
Nervous system, 157
    diseases of, 165
Netelast, 245
Noise, 4
Nose, 50
    bleeding from, 65
    foreign bodies in, 245

Observation of patients, 18
Occipital bone, 183
Odontoid process, 180
Oedema, 20
Oesophagus, 96
Olive oil enema, 31
Operations,
    preparation for, 138
    after care, 139
Ophthalmia neonatorum, 220
Optic nerve, 169
Orchitis, 219
Orthopnoea, 27
Ossicles, 174
Osteo-arthritis, 190
Osteomyelitis, 192
Ovaries, 204
Oxygen,
    administration of, 57
    dangers of, 57

Palate bones, 183
Pancreas, 98
Paralysis, 161
Paraplegia, 161
Parasympathetic nervous system, 160
Parathyroid glands, 117
Parietal bones, 183
Pasteurized milk, 92
Patch test, 217
Patella, 188

Pellagra, 90
Pelvis, 186
Penicillin, 125
Pepsin, 101
Peptic ulcer, 107
Pericarditis, 67
Pericardium, 60
Perineum, 204
Periosteum, 122
Peristalsis, 98
Peritoneum, 100
Peritonitis, 101
Personal hygiene, 2
Petit mal, 166
Phalanges, 186, 188
Pharynx, 96
Phlebitis, 69
Phosphorus, in food, 90
Pia mater, 159
Pink eye, 171
Pinna, 174
Pituitary gland, 115
Plasma, 71
Plaster of Paris, 199
Platelets, 71
Pleura, 52
Pleurisy, 55
Pneumonia, types of, 54
Poisons, 239
Poliomyelitis, 135
Pons varolii, 159
Positions in nursing, 13
Pott's fracture, 198
Poultices, kaolin, 75
    starch, 49
Pressure points, 236
    sores, 42
Prevention of accidents, 230
Prostate gland, 203
Protein, in food, 89
    in urine, 81
Protoplasm, 150
Psoriasis, 47
Ptyalin, 101

Pulmonary arteries, 59
Pulmonary tuberculosis, 216
Pulse, 26
Purpura, 45
Pus, 74
Pustule, 45
Pyelitis, 87
Pyloric stenosis, 107
Pyrexia, 23

Quarantine, 131

Rabies, 128
Radius, 185
Rats, infection from, 128
Recovery tray, 139
Recreation, 1
Rectal washout, 32
Rectum, 98
   examination, 33
Rehabilitation, 208
Rennin, 101
Reproductive system, 202
Respiration, 27
   artificial, 239
Respiratory system, 50
   diseases of, 52
Retention of urine, 79
Retina, 169
Rheumatism, 155
Rheumatoid arthritis, 191
Rhinitis, 53
Ribs, 183
Rickets, 192
Rigor, 24
Rigor mortis, 155
Ringworm, 48
Roughage, 91
Round worms, 29

Sacrum, 179
Salivary glands, 95
Sarcoma, 215
Salt-free diet, 105

Scabies, 47
Scalds, 244
Scapula, 186
Scarlet fever, 134
Sciatica, 167
Scurvy, 91
Sebaceous glands, 36
   cysts, 48
Seborrhaea, 48
Sebum, 36
Sedatives, 125
Septicaemia, 75
Serum, 131
   sickness, 131
Sex glands, 118
Shingles, 166
Shock, 233
Sighing, 27
Skeleton, 177
Skin, 36
   care of, 37
   diseases of, 45
   traction, 199
Skull, 181
Sodium chloride, 90
Sordes, 39
Sound waves, 176
Specific gravity, 78
Sphenoid bone, 183
Spirochaetes, 127
Spleen, 114
Sprains, 198
Sputum, 19
Stapes, 174
Staphylococci, 126
Starch poultice, 49
Stenosis, mitral, 67
   pyloric, 107
Sterilization, 137
Sternum, 183
Stertorous breathing, 27
Stings, 243
Stomach, 96
Stools, 224

Streptococci, 126
Stye, 171
Suffocation, 235
Supplementary feeding, 227
Suppositories, 29
Suppression of urine, 79
Surgical nursing, 136
Sutures of skull, 181
Sweat glands, 36
Sweating, 44
Sympathetic nervous
    system, 160
Synovial membrane, 151
Synovitis, 193
Syphilis, 218
Systole, 70

Tapeworms, 28
Tarsal bones, 188
Teeth, 94
    Hutchinson's, 218
    infants, 223
Temperature, 20
Temporal bones, 183
Tendon of Achilles, 154
Tepid sponging, 25
Testes, 202
Tetany, 156
Thermometers, 21
Thoracic duct, 112
Thorax, bones of, 183
Thread worms, 29
Thrombosis, 69
Thymus gland, 118
Thyroid gland, 116
Thyrotoxicosis, 117
Tibia, 188
Tinea, 48
Tissues, 150
Tourniquet, 238
Toxaemia, 75
Trachea, 51
Traction, 199
Tranquillizers, 125

Trapezius, 153
Triceps, 153
Trypsin, 101
Tubegauz, 245
Tuberculosis, 216
Turbinated bones, 183
Typhoid fever, 135

Ulna, 185
Unconsciousness, 233
Undulant fever, 93
Ureter, 78
Urethra, 78
Urine, 78
    testing of, 80
Urinometer, 79
Uterus, 203

Vaccines, 129
Vagina, 204
Vaginal examination, 205
Vagus nerve, 159
Valuables, care of, 16
Veins, 62
Vena cavae, 59
Venereal disease, 218
Vesicle, 45
Vertebrae, 179
Villi, 98
Viruses, 127
Vitamins, 90
Vitreous humour, 170
Vomer, 183
Vomiting, 19
Vulva, 203

Ward reports, 6
Weaning, 228
Weal, 45
Whooping cough, 133
Worms, 28

Yawning, 27